THE BROOKE
BOOK

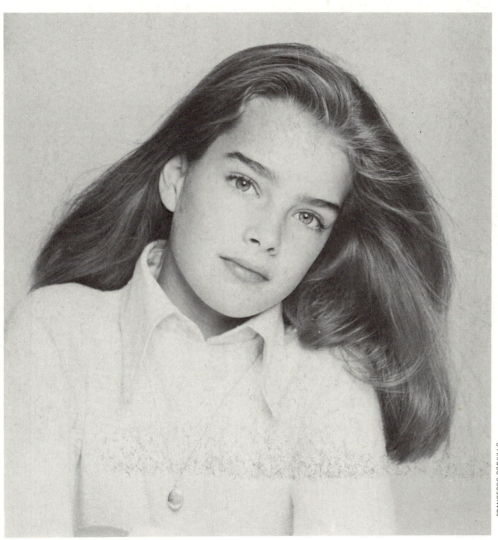

FRANCESCO SCAVULLO

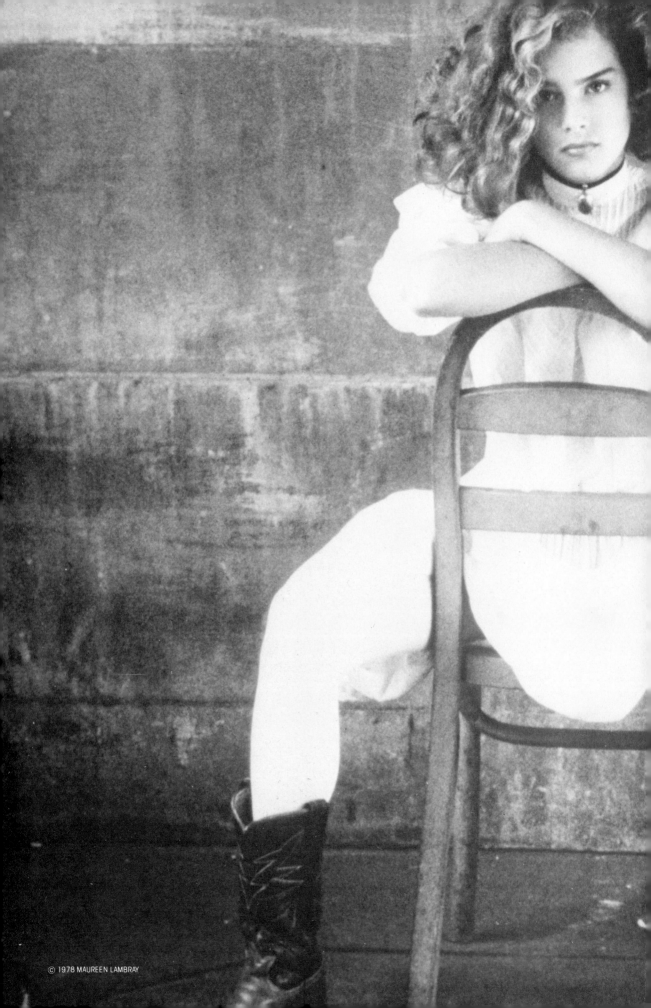

THE BROOKE BOOK

by Brooke Shields

A WALLABY BOOK
PUBLISHED BY POCKET BOOKS NEW YORK

To my momma and all the people who made this book possible.

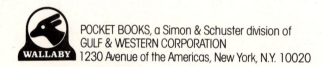
POCKET BOOKS, a Simon & Schuster division of
GULF & WESTERN CORPORATION
1230 Avenue of the Americas, New York, N.Y. 10020

ISBN: 0-671-79018-8

First Wallaby printing March, 1978

Designed by Jacques Chazaud

1   2   9   8

Trademarks registered in the United States and other countries.

Printed in the U.S.A.

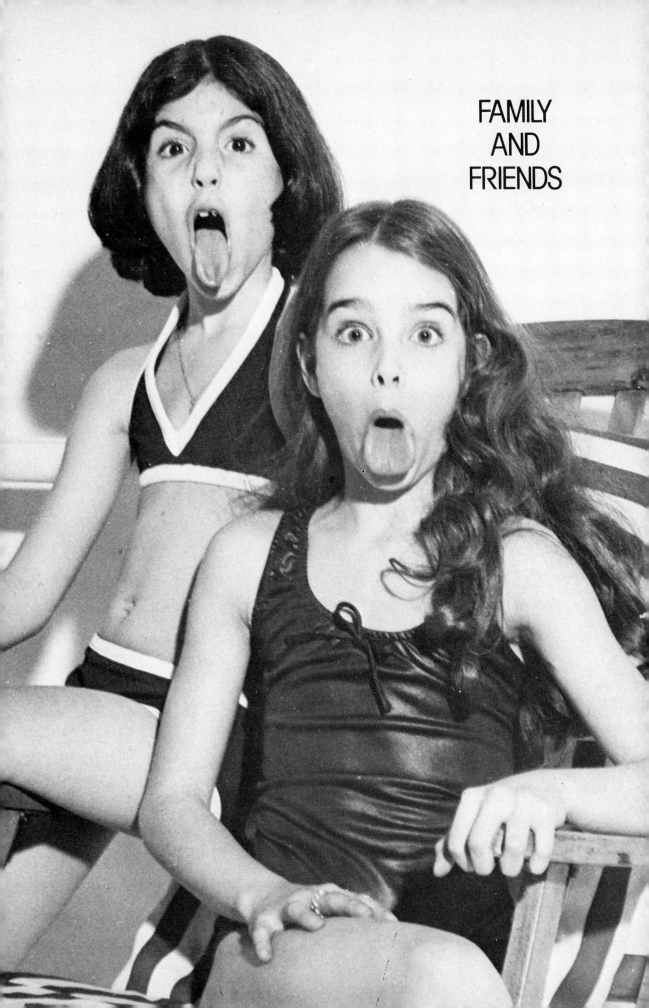

FAMILY
AND
FRIENDS

In the
beginning
there was . . .

       BROOKE

           as of 1965 that is . . .

THE CITY OF NEW YORK – DEPARTMENT OF HEALTH
BUREAU OF RECORDS AND STATISTICS

CERTIFICATE OF BIRTH REGISTRATION
(THIS IS NOT A CERTIFIED COPY. SEE* BELOW)

Certificate of Birth

OF RECORDS
DEPARTMENT OF HEALTH
BOROUGH OF MANHATTAN
FILED

JUN 2 AM 10:38

Certificate No. 156-65-113365

1. Full name of child (PRINT)	BROOKE *First name*	CHRISTA *Middle name*	SHIELDS *Last name*

2. Sex FEMALE	3. Number of children born of this pregnancy 1	5. Date of child's birth (Month) MAY (Day) 31 (Year) 1965	5a. Hour 1:45 P.	
	4. If more than one, number of this child in order of birth			

6. PLACE OF BIRTH
(a) NEW YORK CITY: (b) Borough MANHATTAN
(c) Name of Hospital or Institution NEW YORK POLYCLINIC HOSPITAL
(d) If not in hospital, street address No. .... Ave. St.

7. USUAL RESIDENCE OF MOTHER:
(a) State NEW YORK
(b) Co. NEW YORK (c) City or Town NEW YORK
(d) No. 400 EAST 52ND STREET Ave. St.

FATHER	MOTHER
8. Full name FRANCIS ALEXANDER SHIELDS	12. Full maiden name TERESA ANN SCHMON
9. Age at time of this birth 24 years	13. Age at time of this birth 31 years
10. Birthplace (City or place and State, or Country) NEW YORK	14. Birthplace (City or place and State, or Country) NEW YORK
11a. Usual Occupation PURCHASING AGENT	15a. Total number of children BORN ALIVE PREVIOUS to this pregnancy NONE
11b. Kind of business or industry in which work was done STEEL INDUSTRY	15b. Number of children born PREVIOUS to this pregnancy and NOW LIVING NONE

I hereby certify that this child was born alive at the hour and on the date stated above, and that all the facts stated in this certificate and report of birth are true to the best of my knowledge, information and belief.

Date of Report May 31 1965

Given name added from a supplemental report _____ (Date of) _____
Borough Registrar.

(Signed) H. H. Lardaro
Name of Signer H. H. LARDARO (Print or typewrite)
Address 400 E. 50th St. New York, N.Y.

Print here the mailing address of mother.➡ Copy of this certificate will be mailed to her when it is filed with the Department of Health.

Name MRS. TERESA SHIELDS
Address 400 EAST 52ND STREET Apt.
City NEW YORK Post Office Zone 10022 State NEW YORK

BUREAU OF RECORDS AND STATISTICS   DEPARTMENT OF HEALTH   THE CITY OF NEW YOR

INFORMATION. IF THE CERTIFICATE _____ _____ CORRECT INFORMATION TO THE DIVISION OF RECORDS IN THE BOROUGH WHERE THE CHILD WAS BORN. (SEE ADDRESS BELOW.) YOU WILL BE ADVISED HOW TO HAVE THE RECORD CORRECTED. IT IS IMPORTANT TO DO THIS AT ONCE.

*A COPY BEARING THE RAISED SEAL OF THE DEPARTMENT OF HEALTH MAY BE OBTAINED UPON PAYMENT OF THE REQUIRED FEE WHENEVER IT IS NEEDED FOR OFFICIAL PROOF OF THE FACTS REGARDING THIS BIRTH.

Robert F. Wagner Jr.	George James, M.D.	Carl L. Erhardt, Sc.D.
MAYOR	COMMISSIONER OF HEALTH	DIRECTOR OF BUREAU

MANHATTAN: 125 WORTH STREET   BROOKLYN: 295 FLATBUSH AVENUE EXTENSION
THE BRONX: 1826 ARTHUR AVENUE   QUEENS: 90-37 PARSONS BOULEVARD, JAMAICA
RICHMOND: 51 STUYVESANT PLACE, ST. GEORGE, S.I.

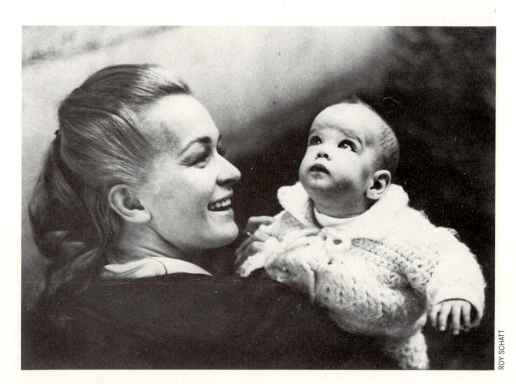

A few of the 4000 pictures my mommy bought.

A POEM FOR MOTHER

Mothers are good
     but you're the best one.
No other person could have won . . .
     the trophy I won . . . for having
You as a mother.

                    1974

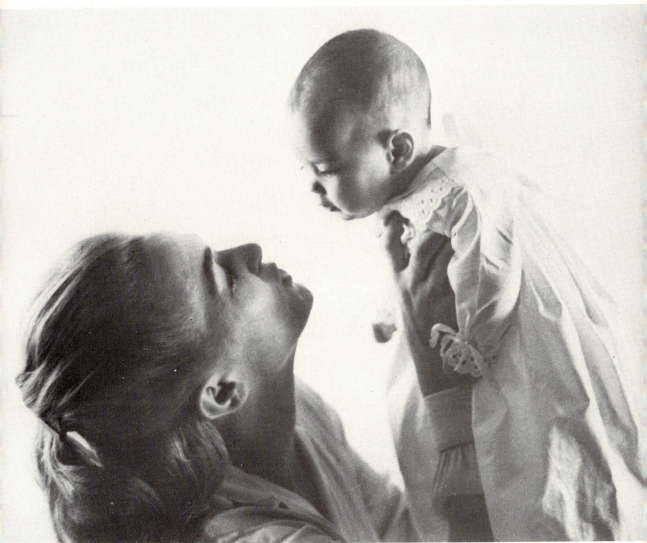

ROY SCHATT

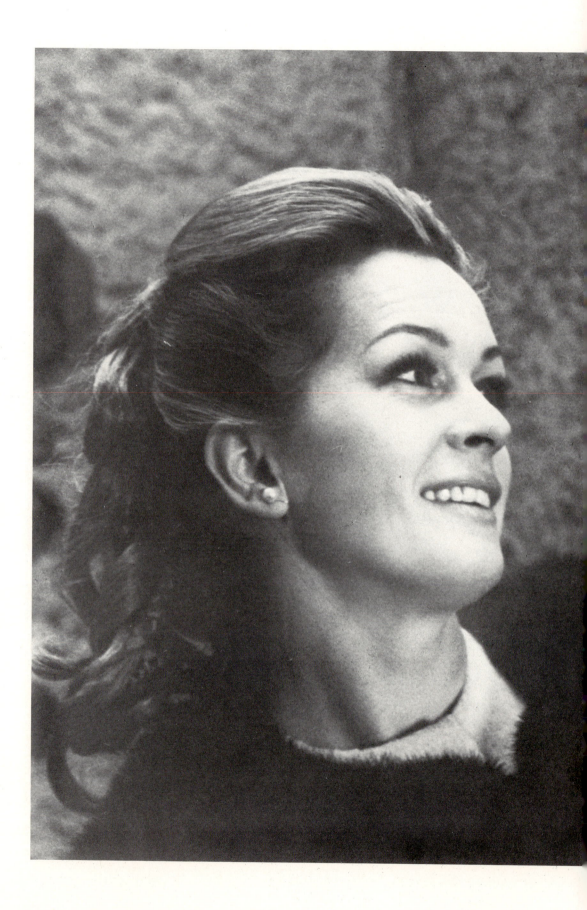

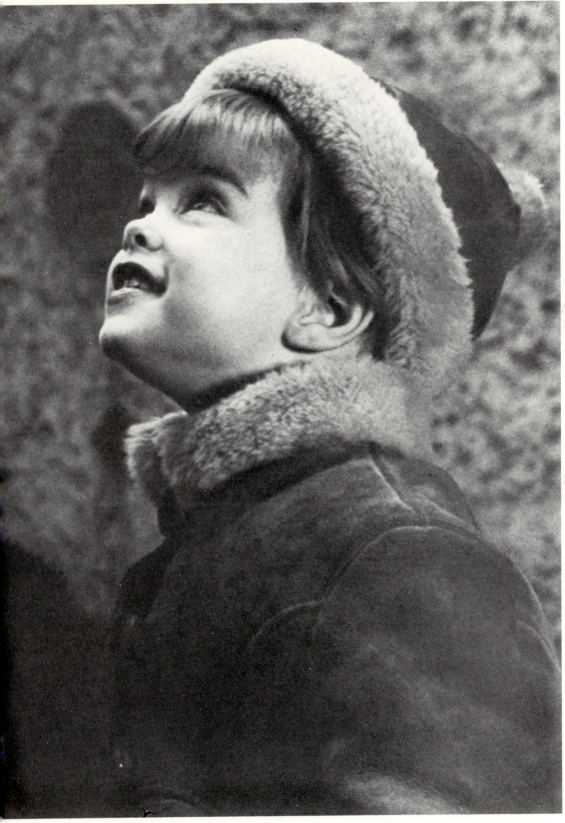

I was born on a Monday afternoon at 1:45 on May 31, 1965. I almost arrived in the back seat of my daddy's car. We all made it to the hospital just in time. I arrived two months early. I weighed five pounds, three ounces and was a foot and a half tall. My features were absolutely beautiful and the nurses said I was a perfect pink.

I was a good baby but I cried alot because I had colic which is a very bad stomach ache. Other than that I was a healthy baby.

My eating habits were strange. I refused all my food except my bottle. My mother decided to put all my food in my bottle, so she made the hole in the nipple larger. It contained milk, cereal, vitamins, fruit and sugar. Then I decided to give the bottle up for hot dogs. That lasted until I was two years old. From that time on I decided to eat everything.

At the age of seven months I tried walking. My mother noticed that my feet looked like they were on the wrong legs. The doctor corrected the problem and I was walking at eleven months.

My first words were no, dada, mama, very dangerous and I'm serious. At this age, which was about a year old, I would hail taxis for my mother. I would put my hand up and shout, "SIR." I also started modeling at this point in my life.

During my first year of life I received my first two teeth. When I was three months old my mother recalls rubbing my gums while she was on the phone, she screamed. Her friend thought there was something wrong but my mother was screaming with happiness to have discovered my first teeth. I didn't get any more after that until I was almost one. The doctor thought it was very strange.

I never liked to go to sleep (still don't). When I was really tiny my mom would force my head down and I would pop it up. We would take turns until my head became so heavy it would drop with a thud. I guess that's the only bad habit I have.

I have always talked alot. When I was very small I would say, dat-dat-dat in my crib. For hours I

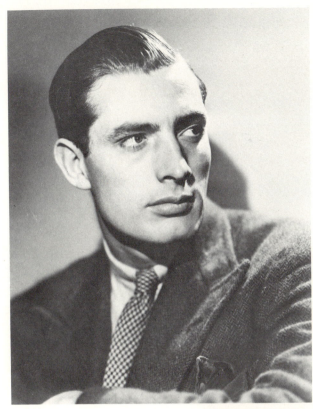

Pop Pop. A winning tennis champ.

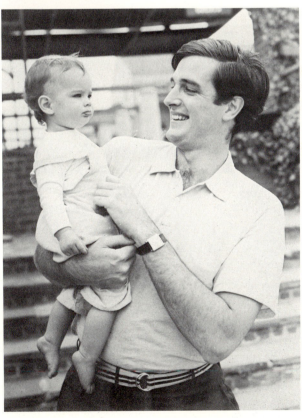

July 4th weekend with my father. 1966

wouldn't shut up. I'd say it loud then very softly, then fast, followed by an angry tone, and at last falling asleep.

My mom recalls an incident in the hospital. It seems that an annoying squeak kept all the new mothers awake. Mom spoke up and asked if the squeaky door could be fixed. The nurse told my mother that all that squeak needed was a warm bottle and attention. Sure enough that squeak was little me, so I guess I've been babbling all my life. That is also how I kind of got my name, Babbling Brooke.

Another incident Mom remembers was one day I was on an elevator and there was a lady with her little baby in a stroller. I turned to my mommy and said, "Oh, what a darling baby Ma Ma." The baby's mother was so surprised, "How old are you?" she asked. "Two and a half," I answered in my best British accent. Much to her surprise again she repeated, "Oh, my, just two and a hahf?" "No" I said, "Not two and a hahf . . .two and a half."

I started school when I was four. The school was really terrific and fun. I always asked for homework like the big kids had but now that I get so much, I realize that I must have been a dumb kid with a BIG MOUTH! I loved school then and I especially love it now.

I remember a boy named Drew who would always hit and annoy me and make me cry. I told my mother about him and she said, "Well, if he doesn't stop, make a hard fist and sock him square in the nose." I tried this the next day but I missed his nose and made his chin click. He cried and didn't say a word or bother me for days. Then one morning Drew came to school and handed me a beautiful diamond ring that belonged to his mother. I showed my mom and she gave it back to the teacher. From then on he would sit real real close to me and be quiet and stroke my hair. I didn't like Drew and I do not know what was better, being bopped or loved by him!

Unfortunately the school closed because I think someone ran off with all the school's monies. It was,

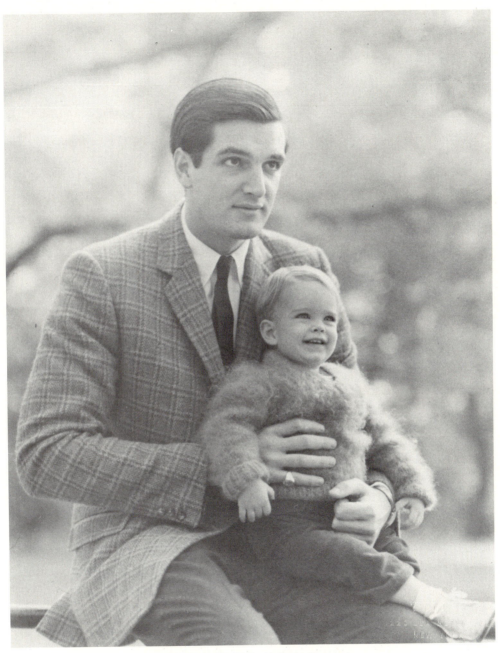

Ciao! Daddy. It's Holly-Holly-Hollywood.

I put my fathers toothbrush next to mine. (1st grade)

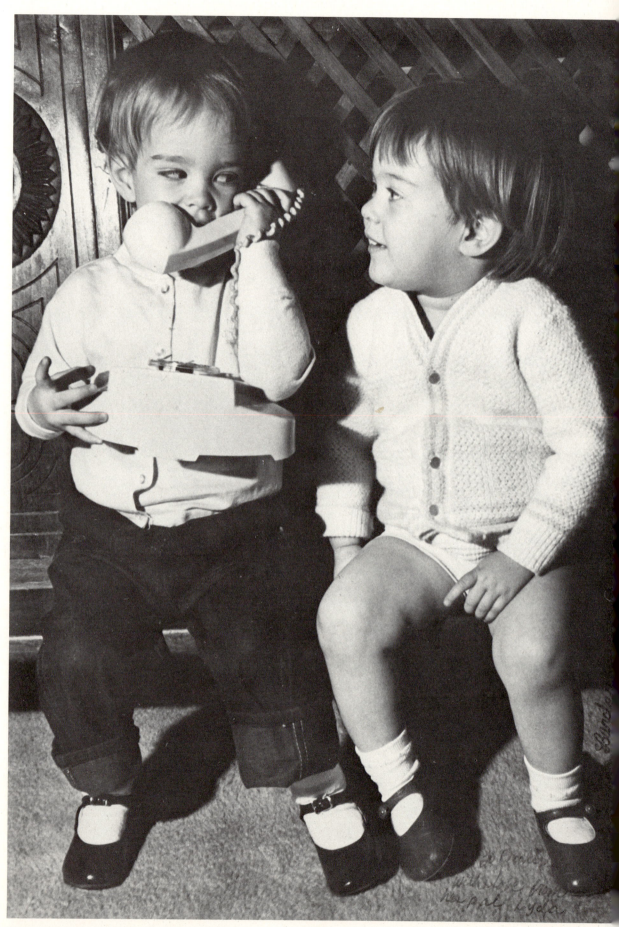

Thanks for the telephone, Lydia. March, 1967.

SUSAN BARCLAY ELY

Lydia, please hang up.
March, 1977.

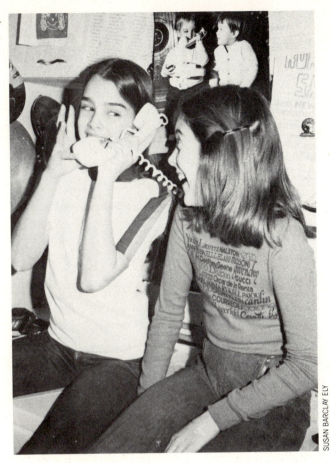

in a way, good for me because I was able to come to Lenox.

I spent most of my summers in Southampton just playing. We became tired of that so we went to Brazil when I was four. Brazil is so beautiful and happy, I didn't want to come home. We met so many wonderful people there and I still get homesick for them at times. I'm planning to go back soon.

I went to Mexico the next year but for some reason I don't remember the trip much other than I had a good time swimming all day. My Mother said I became deathly sick and the doctor who took care of me fell in love with my mother. Mommy sprained her ankle dancing and the doctor carried her all over Mexico. I had to walk. He followed us back to New York but we were not interested. (I was glad.)

The next summer I went to St. Croix on a job for Simplicity Patterns. I was booked for three weeks. I worked two hours the second day and the rest of my time was free. Boy did I have fun.

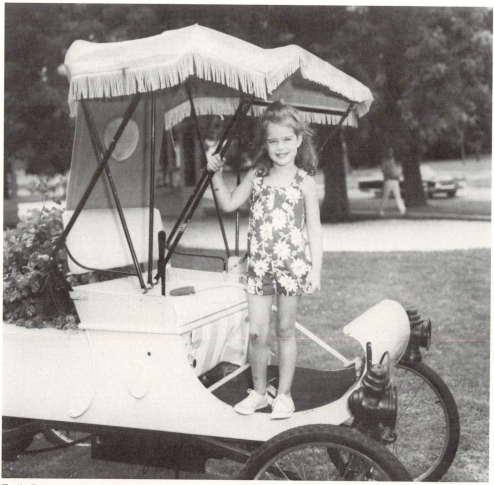

Teri's Tavern of the Erwin House.

We worked our way north to Florida and went to a rodeo and saw Roy Rogers and Dale Evans. I asked for her autograph and because I thought it was proper I gave her mine. We visited Cape Kennedy and saw how all the rockets are made. Then we went to Christmas, Florida, to an alligator farm. Then we came home.

I really love my work because it gives me an opportunity to do alot of things I ordinarily would not be able to do. The money I make also helps with my school and all other activities I want to do.

Right now I'm taking piano lessons and I go to a dance class twice a week. I have joined a tennis club.

I've wanted to learn how to play tennis since I was a little girl. I also go horseback riding every Saturday. Lessons are fun and I get to give the horse some treats, such as carrots or apple biscuits.

I have many friends. Some live far away and I write to them. Most of them are in school.

I love school. My favorite subjects are Math and English. When I think of it, I really love all my subjects. The days are well put together and interesting. The only thing I don't like about school is the two and half hours of gym, straight. I feel it takes me away from my other work. It just seems to drag out the day too long and because it's the first thing in the morning it puts me in a bad mood and I seem to take it out on others. As far as homework is concerned I think we get too much. It takes away from my home life and free time.

My bad habits are few. One of them is sucking my thumb. I only do it when I'm tired or in distress, so it's not really very often.

I remember one time when I really was very young, I told a little boy who was on T.V. to put his thumb in his mouth because a crook was after him. I don't do these kookie things anymore.

The other bad habit is not wanting to go to bed and not wanting to get up. Since my 1977 New Year's Resolution my room is looking better and I'm proud of it when I have friends visit.

I have many hobbies such as swimming, sewing, coloring magazines and coloring photos in a special way a photographer taught me.

Another hobby is that I especially love collecting small items. I love little wooden toys. I have a good collection of them. I feel the things I collect might be collectors' items in the years to come.

Some of the fun things I like to do is helping people in my building. For example, baby sitting (because I love babies), walking dogs and running errands. I get paid a fair price. I also water plants for people who are on vacation. I like going to my friend Bob's office because I get to play secretary with my own office, phone, desk, and even a Xerox machine.

In 1977, January actually, Louis Malle, the French director selected me for the leading role in "Pretty Baby." I was really surprised. Playing Violet was an educational experience and I fell in love with old New Orleans.

Then on October 30th, I became "Tilt" for director Rudy Durand. We arrived in picturesque Santa Cruz, California. The Hollywood crew gave me my wish, a Halloween party. Everyone was in costumes. About two hundred people came. I surprised them all by greeting them as a pinball machine.

In the film, also titled "Tilt," I always win at playing pinball, that's why my name is Tilt. It was fun because they gave me a pinball machine to use and they made a special one for me to keep for my very own in New York. The movie will be out this spring.

Well now I'm off to Canada for "Morning, Winter and Night" but more about that later . . .

As for my future, I intend to continue modeling because I really love it. I will be able to continue my career in that field until it's time to think about getting married. I'd like to have as many children as God allows me to have. I know my family will understand that my career is important to me and that I will be a good wife and mother and not neglect them.

One of my dreams is to be on Broadway. Everytime I see a new musical it encourages me even more. I get a wonderful feeling that I want to get up on the stage with the performers and dance forever.

I'd like to have a brownstone in New York. I'll be doing alot of business in the city and I really love it.

I'd also like to have a house in the country for weekends and the summer. I guess it should be sort of like a farm. I'd like a few animals at first and then build up to alot, gradually. When we are traveling or in New York there will be someone to take care of things.

These are some of my dreams for the future. I hope they come true.

The End

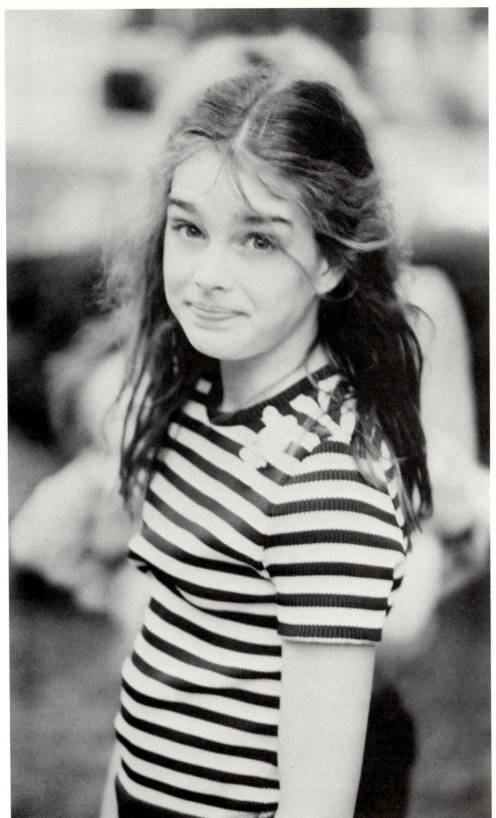

SEVEN

Once upon a time there was a seven.
This seven found a seven and that
seven found a seven but that seven
found a three, and that three found
a three but that three found a two.
This two found a zero. Now this zero
didn't find anything because zeros
are the end. So this is the end.

MOMMY'S TEARS

I woke up in the middle of the night and heard my mother crying in the kitchen. I asked what was wrong. "There is no more time," she said. No more time for what I asked? "No more time to shop! It's eleven o'clock and tomorrow is Christmas."

I knew my mother felt bad because every Christmas she likes to buy the orphans something for the occasion and also, she loves to have big dinner parties. So I said why don't we call the orphanage and our dinner guests and say we are changing the party to Tuesday, two days after Christmas. This way we have a whole day to shop.

Now our problems were solved. Mommy's tears were gone and I felt better, too. When the time came to give the orphans their gifts, it felt like another small Christmas, and our dinner party was a success.

September, 1975

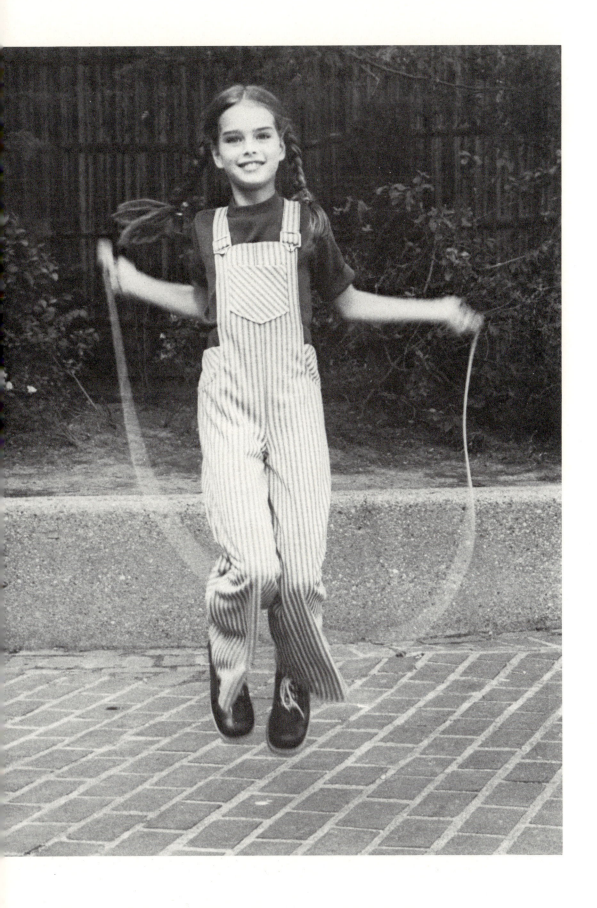

HOW HALLOWEEN GOT STARTED

Once long long ago in a town called Tunesville there was an old abandoned house which everyone said was haunted and had ghosts. No one ever dared to go inside.

There were two ghosts that lived in the house named Harry and Weeny. Harry's friends called him Hallow because he was dumb and had a hollow brain. Weeny's mother named him Weeny because he was the smallest baby in the family.

One day on Friday the 31st of October, Hallow and Weeny were sitting around the house talking about what they were going to do. Hallow got an idea. The idea was for both of the ghosts to go scaring people. So Hallow and Weeny went haunting and scaring people having an absolute ball. When they arrived home they were so tired that they went straight to bed without washing their sheets.

In the morning they decided that they would continue their haunting every year because they had had so much fun the night before.

They decided that they should name their holiday. They thought and thought and then Weeny said, "Why don't we name it after us. Halloweeny."

That's how we got the name Halloween.

The Beginning 1976

I became a flower child.

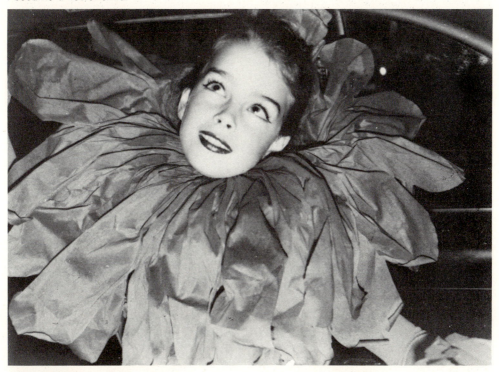

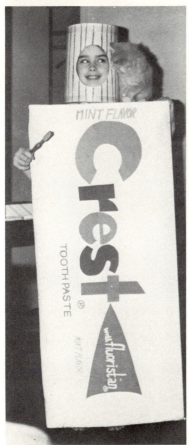

Another Halloween, artwork by Mom.

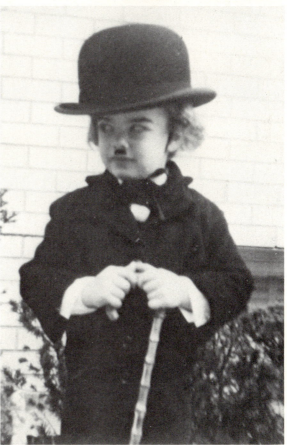

I was Charlie Chaplin 10 years ago.

Brooke Shields
Received for the first time the most sacred Body and
Blood
        of our Lord Jesus Christ
this 8th day of May in the year of our Lord and Savior
1973 in the church of St. Thomas More . . . James
Wilders, pastor.

I want to thank God for everything that he made
especially
        for Jesus in holy communion, let us pray to the
Lord. Brooke

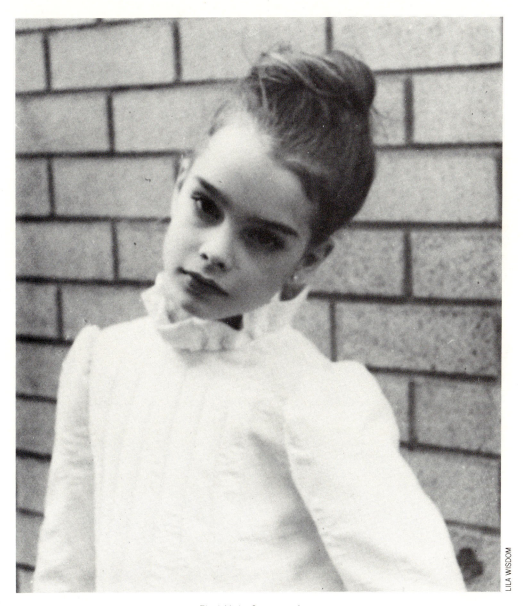

First Holy Communion.

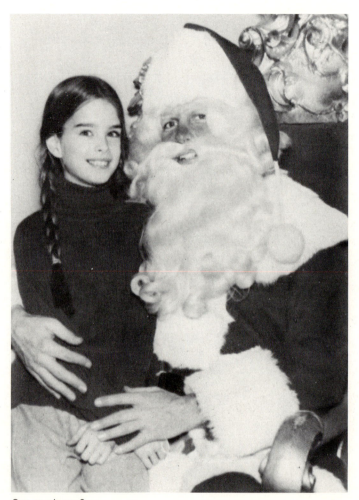

Oscar, please?

I like it for me
I like it for you
I like it for me
But, I like it for you
Especially.

     Baby Brooke (5 years old)

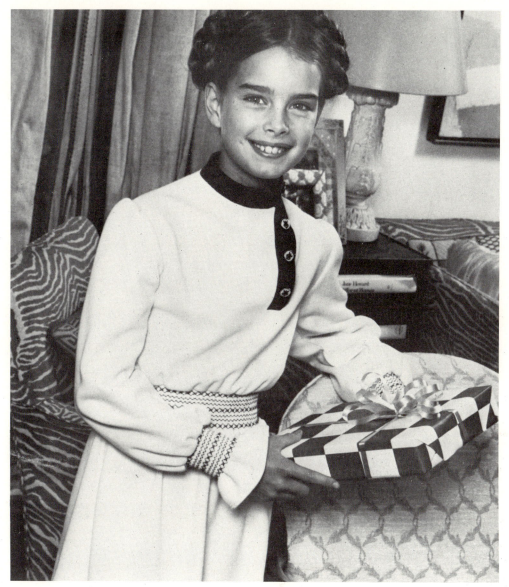

Here I am as Heidi.

TO MY MOMMY

I hope this valentines day
is the best yet
just the same as all the rest.

I love you, I love you,
yes I do
more than anyone
ever knew.

As much as we quarrel
as much as we fight
I love you the same
all day and all night.

I Love You

1976

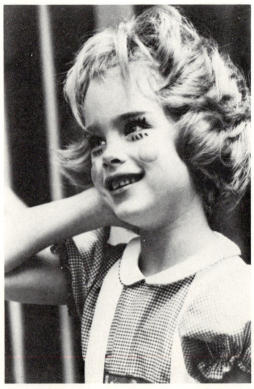

My first Halloween. I was a street cat.

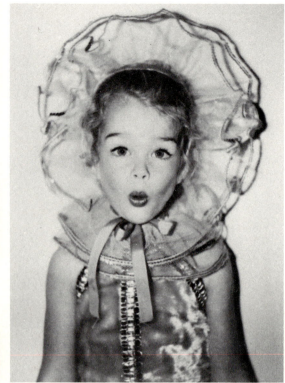

I was a princess for my Carnegie Hall debut.

In 1973, I put on my tap shoes . . .

In Old Tucson

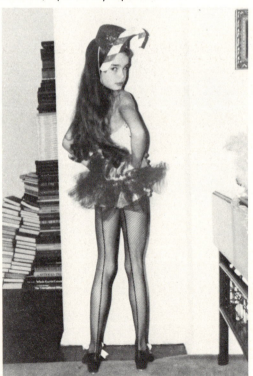

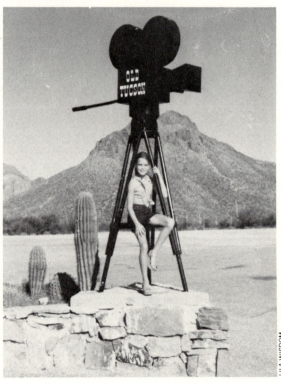

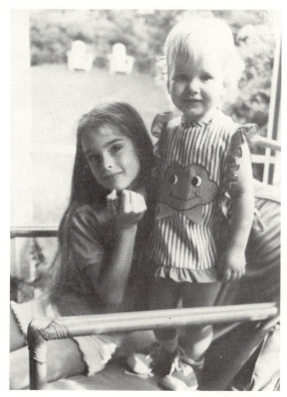

With Baby Sister

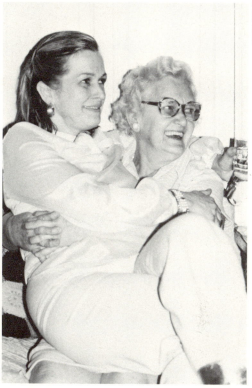

Mom and Grandma

My Long Island family: Christy, the dog, Tommy, Diana, me, Mariana, Christiana, and Jingles the cat.

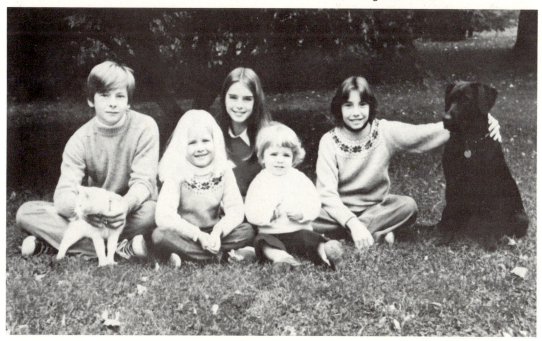

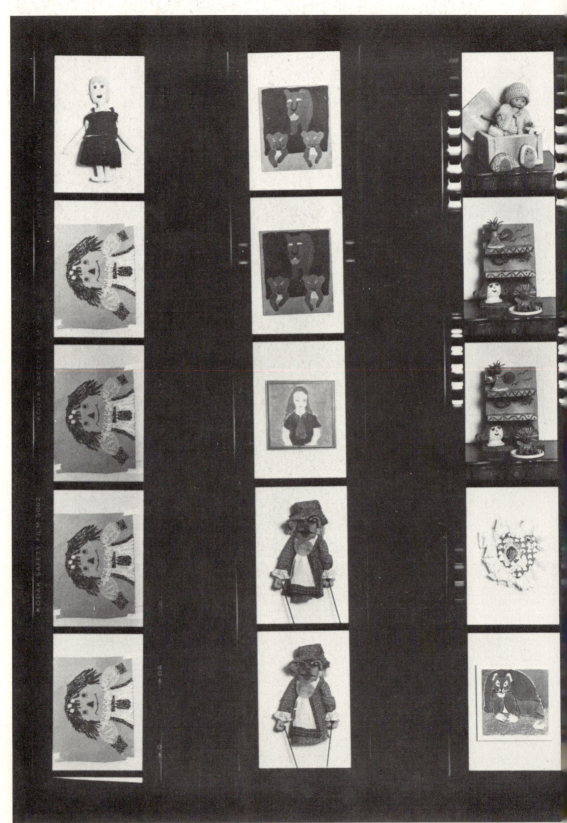

STEVE MILLS

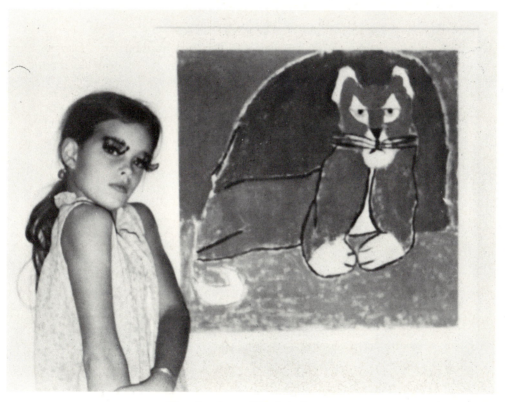

My artwork . . . Mom's lashes.

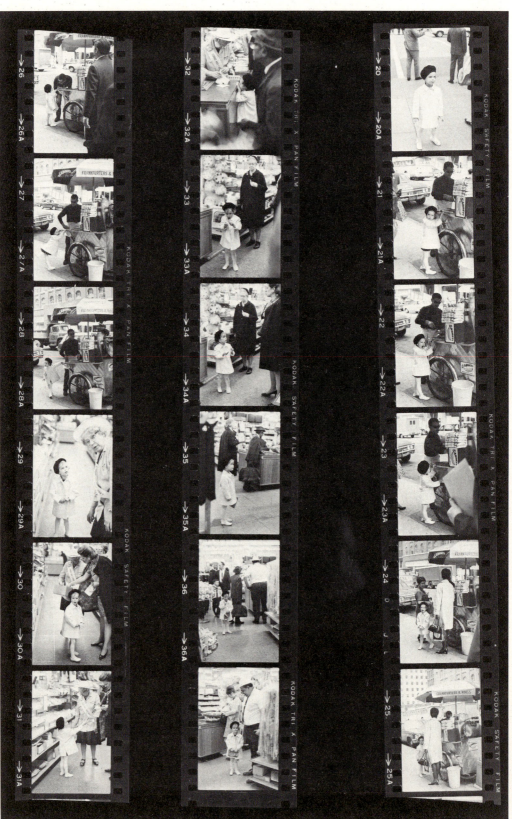

A million-dollar baby . . .

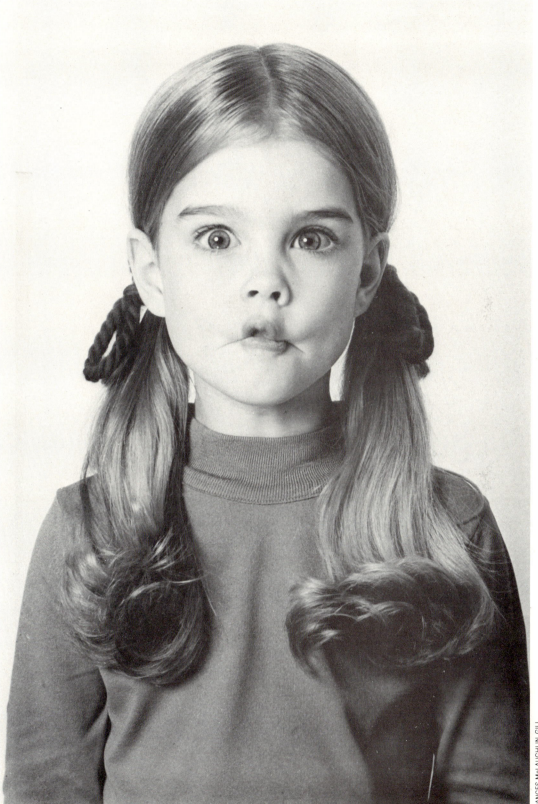

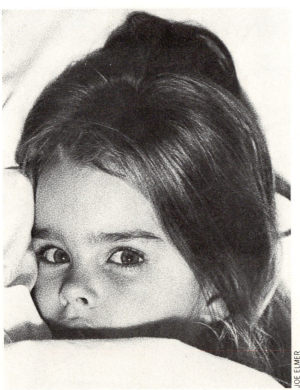
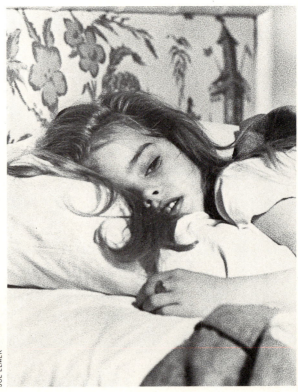

I like going to bed late but
I do not like getting up early.

BEDTIME

Bedtime is a time for rest
    which means a lot of quiet
But sometimes I can't cope
    with it or even can I buy
It when I finally fall asleep
    I dream of things up high
And sometimes I dream that I could fly
    but when I wake up early
I find that night is gone
    then get up ready for school
At the crack of dawn.

1975

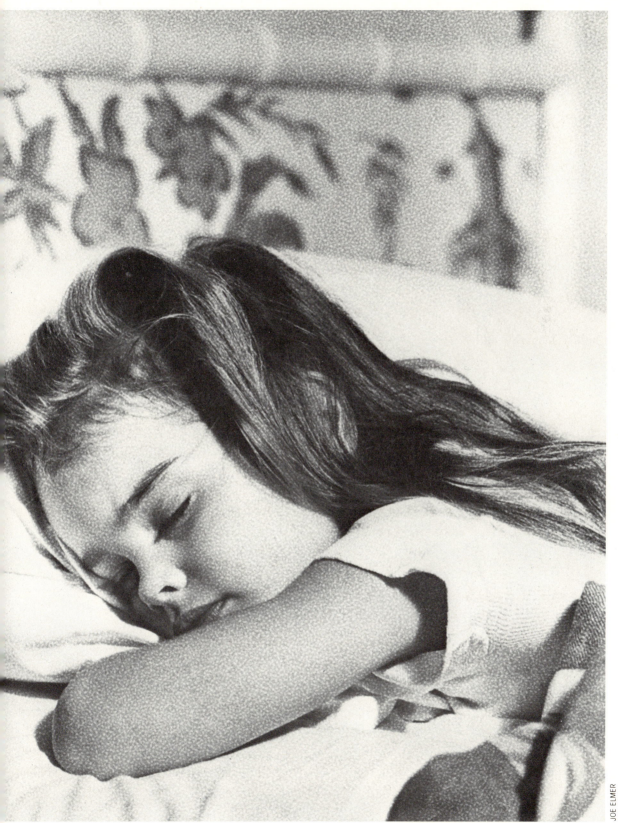

EXCUSES FOR NOT DOING YOUR HOMEWORK

This book is dedicated to all the children who hate homework and need excuses to tell their teachers.

Dear children, I am Mr. Arthur H. Beattie and I am going to tell many different excuses to get away with not doing your homework. This is what you say to your teacher.

1. I was doing my homework on the floor and my mom vacuumed it up.

2. My mom was giving herself a permanent and there were not enough papers to wrap her hair in so she used my homework paper to do it.

3. My dog was being bad so we sent her to obedience school. I started to do my homework when I realized all my pencils had disappeared. That evening my dog's teacher called and said my dog was the best pupil in school because she was ready for school the first day and she brought all her pencils. She must be the teacher's pet.

4. My brother hit me in the face with his baseball bat and he broke my glasses so I became instantly cross-eyed and my vision center wasn't open, so I couldn't do my homework.

5. I was climbing up to my tree house and I fell off and landed on my writing fingers.

6. We went to Africa and a hippo stepped on my paper.

7. My brother had his radio on too loud and my ears were paralyzed, therefore I could not hear myself think.

8. I was walking home from school when I spotted a dollar, so I put two hands on it so no-one would say, "Oh, that's mine." When I started to pick it up someone stepped on my fingers and crushed them so I could not write.

9. When termites were spreading, they came into my room first and ate all my pencils.

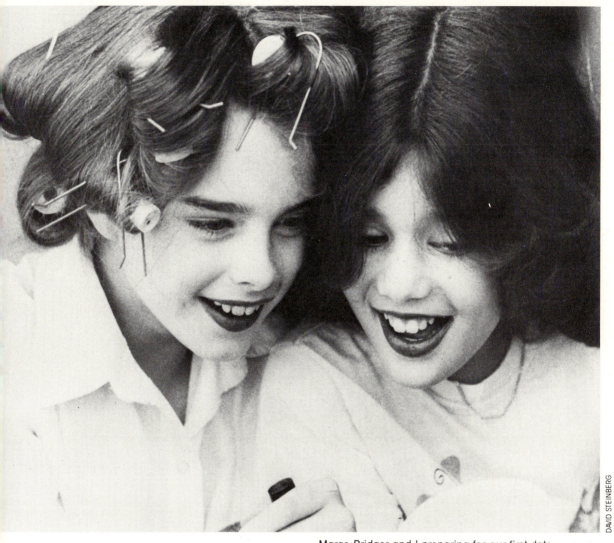

DAVID STEINBERG

Margo Bridger and I preparing for our first date.

10.   My mom was making a pattern and she needed paper so she used my homework.

11.   My father put all my money into the toilet so I couldn't buy any utensils for homework.

12.   I was reading a National Geographic book when I read give all paper to be recycled so I did it and that was my good deed for the day.

13.   My dog didn't like me doing my homework and not playing with her so she ate all of it.

14.   My friend took a picture of me with a million-watt bulb and dots of different colors came in front of my eyes so I couldn't see my homework.

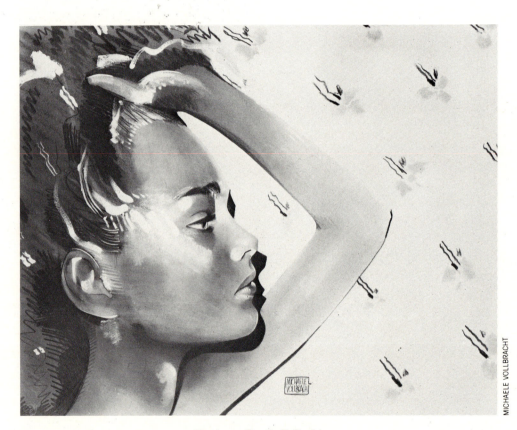

The Lone Star Café Sketch

T & S

Hewwo my dame is Tallulah and I amb five years ode, I am goin do dill you about Febrary fourtimph. Bwell, it all sparted when I woked up. I woked up at tebn ocwok, I got dreffed, ate and went do kool. I had awedy made ma vawentines and oh, I amost fogot, there is a very cute boy in ma class damed Stewie. To I got do kool earwy so we could twade vawentines. I walked up do Stewie and I said, "Stewie" and he said, "yes" and I said, "I don't kave a vawentine for you", and he said, "I don't kave a vawentine for you", and he said, "come over here", so I bwent and he said, "I have one for you Tallulah" and I said "Stewie, I really had one for you to." Se we exganghed them and I dave him a diss on de cheek and I had the bet day at kool in ma hole wife.

The End

COMMENTS

Brooke is self possessed, objective, with emotions that are kept well under control. She is ruled by her head rather than her heart. It is important for her to have the feeling of security in all she does. She will act with good judgment, and even in emergencies will look at alternate courses.

Problems and pressures will bother her and will have a lasting affect on her personality. In times of stress instead of expressing her intense feelings (the way she really feels) she has repressed them. She may have an occasional outburst as a release for these repressions.

She is a careful, slow thinker making sure she has all the facts on hand. She has the ability to get her own information "first-hand". She has the ability to analyze the information she has obtained.

Her goals are set in the practical area with strong willpower and good determination to see them through Her desire to acquire and her openmindedness are forces that will help her achieve her goals.

Her emotional insecurity has bred fear:
Jealously - fear of any rivalry (may spur her on)
Desire for attention - If she is on center stage she will receive all the attention and love that she needs.
Sensitivity to Criticism - Fear of disapproval. She is able to hide these fears from the view of others. (also can spur her on to achievement)

Brooke will try to hold on strongly to that which she believes in (tenacious) and has the propensity to argue (if just to prove a point)

She has good color sense and can work creatively with her hands.

She is good with details, can make decisions and enjoys change in her life. She can be trusted with confidential information and is a good listener.

A New Slant

Graphoanalysis Profile

Personality assessment through the science of handwriting analysis

PERSONALITY PROFILE OF:

BROOKE SHIELDS

PREPARED BY:

SHEILA KURTZ

DATE:

NOVEMBER 1977

SHEILA KURTZ

*This profile analysis pinpoints the most significant personality and motivational traits. It was prepared following the principles of **GRAPHOANALYSIS**, the scientific system of handwriting analysis.*

EMOTIONAL MAKE-UP

☐ Withdrawn—self interest
☒ Poised, objective, uses judgment
☐ Emotionally responsive—tempered by objectivity
☐ Highly responsive, impulsive

HOW EMOTIONAL EXPERIENCES AFFECT YOU

☐ Surface emotions, easily forgotten
☒ Deep emotions, long remembered

MENTAL PROCESSES

☐ Keen comprehension; quick perceptive thinker
☐ Analytical; reasoning ability
☐ Exploratory; investigates data
☒ Careful, slow; builds one fact upon another

IMAGINATION

☐ Ability to penetrate into abstract areas
☐ Area of creative action

GOALS

☐ Unrealistic, day dreams
☐ Ambitious
☒ Practical
☐ Limited

X☒ Willpower
☒ Determination

SOCIAL TRAITS

X	Conservative
	Deceptiveness
	Dignity
	Diplomacy
	Directness
	Domineering
	Enthusiasm
	Frankness
X	Generosity
	Humor
	Impatience, Irritability
	Intuitive
	Loner
	Physical Minded
	Pride
XX	Reticence
	Rhythm
	Sarcasm
X	Secretive
	Self Consciousness
	Selfishness
X	Sensitivity
	Stubborn
	Temper
	Vanity

FORCES TO ACHIEVE

X	Acquisitive
	Aggressive
X	Attention to Details
	Broadminded
	Caution
	Concentration
	Confusion of Interests
XX	Decisive
	Defiant
X	Desires Change & Variety
	Desires Responsibility
	Fluidity
	Independent Thinker
	Initiative
X	Manual Dexterity
	Organizational Ability
	Persistence
X	Positive
	Procrastination
	Resentment
	Self Confidence
	Shallowness
X	Tenacity
	Yieldingness

FEARS

X	Desire for Attention
alert	Jealousy
X	Repression
	Self Castigation
	Self Underestimation

CULTURAL

X	Color Sense
X	Creativity
	Line Appreciation
	Literary Leanings
	Showmanship

My favorite type of horse is
the Bay because they are very beautiful.
Bay has a brown body and a black
mane and tail,
                        Love
                        Brooke Shields

HOROSCOPE CHART

Success at a young age and international fame are the two outstanding factors in Brooke Shields birth chart. At the time of her birth, Jupiter, the planet of Greater Good Fortune, and the sun were exactly in the same position in the sign of Gemini. A few degrees away was the planet of luck, beauty, love and money — Venus — close to the Moon's position, also in Gemini. Being born on the New Moon, while having the additional luck and support of these other planets of fortune, whatever Brooke was to do would zoom her into the limelight.

This powerful grouping of planets at the top of her chart emphasized, first, a major career success when the planet Jupiter returned to its original position (it takes 12 years to do so) and triggered off the luck, as well as the benefits of the rest of the planets, one by one. The aspects from the other planets to this celestial conjunction look like spotlights keeping her in the public eye and supporting her talents both with luck and ease, and also with diligence and hard work. Brooke is now entering her big career period despite the great success already achieved. She is destined to be one of the great stars of the world, and while she may have to bear the burden of hard work and fame at an early age, she will develop the wisdom and philosophy that will enable her to handle all obstacles and enjoy the rewarding personal life and stardom that she is destined to have bestowed upon her.

BROOKE SHIELDS.

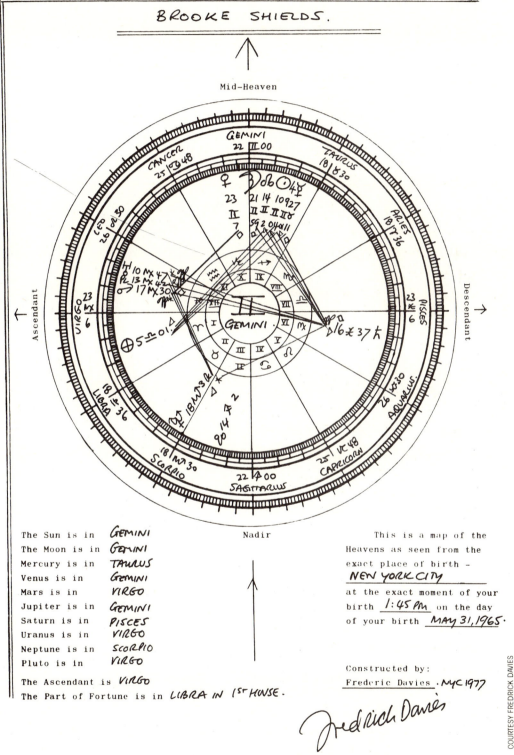

Mid-Heaven

Ascendant

Descendant

Nadir

The Sun is in *GEMINI*
The Moon is in *GEMINI*
Mercury is in *TAURUS*
Venus is in *GEMINI*
Mars is in *VIRGO*
Jupiter is in *GEMINI*
Saturn is in *PISCES*
Uranus is in *VIRGO*
Neptune is in *SCORPIO*
Pluto is in *VIRGO*

The Ascendant is *VIRGO*
The Part of Fortune is in *LIBRA IN 1ST HOUSE.*

This is a map of the Heavens as seen from the exact place of birth – *NEW YORK CITY* at the exact moment of your birth *1:45 PM* on the day of your birth *MAY 31, 1965.*

Constructed by:
Frederic Davies . *NYC 1977*

Fredrich Davies

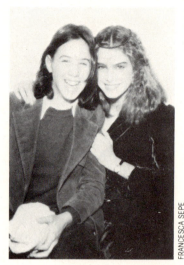

My friend Merrill in a loft in Soho.
We were testing Lucrezia Borgia
for Danelle Sentore.

FRANCESCA SEPE

BROOKE INTERVIEWING A FRIEND

Brooke: What are you going to name your child if it's a
girl?
Friend: I think her name is Louise, or, ah, or I don't
know.
What if it's a boy?
John Adams, that's his first name.
What other names do you have picked out if
it's a boy?
Oh, I don't know if I have enough money to
make the expenses, for crying out loud, you
know you could have better questions, now,
come on. I would like to look for dimes.
Well, if you stay a little while I'll give you two
dollars.
O.K., ask me any questions you want, honey.
Alright now, where do you shop for your
clothes?
I make my own clothes and sometimes I find
them in the garbage cans, you know.
You must be very talented.
Yea, you gotta be talented in my life, honey.
This has been a very nice interview, I hope to
see you again.
Give me my two dollars and I want to leave.
Good-by, I hope you enjoyed the interview.

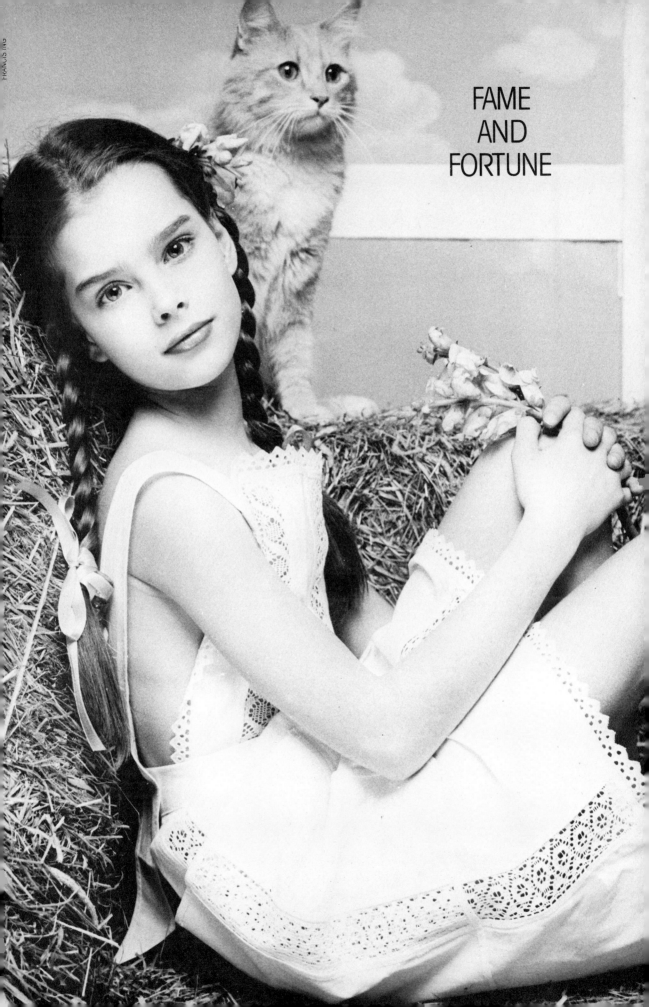

FAME
AND
FORTUNE

FORD MODELS, INC.

344 East 59th St., New York, New York 10022
Murray Hill 8-8538
Telex 224443 - Chevy

April, 1975

Hello . . . .

    We at Ford are very enthusiastic
about a new, rising star named BROOKE SHIELDS.

    BROOKE has an I.Q. of 155. . . a
photographic memory. . . and total recall.
Never a problem with lines or scripts.

    BROOKE is <u>exclusive</u> with FORD! You
may reach her by calling FORD CHILDREN and
asking for Claudia.

    Thank you,

    FORD CHILDREN'S DIVISION

A RISING STAR
By Eugenia Sheppard

Though Brooke Shields was just 12 years old on her last birthday, May 31, she has already written her autobiography, and the things that have happened to her in that short time more than justify the story.

The autobiography, along with some of her poems, will be included in "The Brooke Book," along with advertisements she has posed for and stills from movies in which she had parts.

Compiled by John Holland, a friend of the family, it will be published in an oversize paperback by Pocket Books (Wallaby) next spring timed for the opening of the Louis Malle film, "Pretty Baby," in which Brooke will have star billing for the first time.

Brooke is the daughter of notoriously handsome, 6-foot-7, Revlon vice president Frank Shields and his first wife, Teri, an attractive ex-model.

Her grandfather on the Shields side was Francis X. Shields, whose name was synonymous with tennis, and her grandmother was Princess Marina Torlonia, an international beauty. To go back even further, her great-grandmother was Olivia Moore of Boston, who went to Europe and married Italian Prince Torlonia in the days when girls didn't do such daring things.

"Sometimes I think I look like my grandmother, but I know I look like my father. I think he worries about what I'm doing, but I don't quite know why," Brooke said this week at Maureen Lambrey's photo studio.

She was wearing a shirt and jeans and sitting remarkably still as hair stylist Francois gave her pigtail pin curls.

Brooke was photographed for the first time by Francesco Scavullo when she was 7 months old as an Ivory soap baby.

When she was 8 she had a small part in a movie, and at 10 she was a little girl in "A Prince in the Park," which had Ruth Gordon in the cast.

In between, her delicate, expressive little face became familiar in the advertisements for children's clothes.

My first job,
for Ivory with Lisa Palmer.
February, 1967.

For young looking skin
like this

Nothing's more important
than Ivory's purity and
mildness.

FRANCESCO SCAVULLO

"Lots of scripts are sent to us. My mother and I read all of them together and discuss them. I turned down 'Jaws' because I was supposed to be a 15-year-old girl who got eaten by a shark, and I didn't like the idea," she said yesterday.

She has just come back from New Orleans where she spent three months for the filming of "Pretty Baby."

"I'm the pretty baby," she said.

"It's a turn-of-the-century picture. I wear long black stockings and high button shoes. The story is all about a house of prostitutes, and in the end I become one. Doing the part was quite a lot of fun."

When she left New York for New Orleans with the cast and director Louis Malle, Brooke was just a little girl carrying a doll, but when she returned, she had added a couple of inches and looked like a teenager.

The doll had been stuffed into the bottom of a basket, John Holland observed.

Besides acting, which she likes best, and writing, which comes second, Brooke is attracted to art.

"I make sculptures out of dough and I like to paint." She also went to ballet classes for four years, plays the piano and "I'd like to learn to sing, but I may have to wait a little bit."

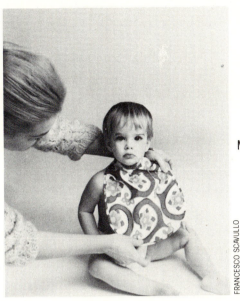

FRANCESCO SCAVULLO

My second job.

This year she is changing schools from Lenox to the new Lincoln, where she will enter seventh grade.

"I don't have any trouble doing both school work and fitting in my jobs. I just tell the school ahead of time and its easy to catch up. In Lenox my friends grew along with me and didn't feel there was anything unusual about my life. In the new school they may be more likely to notice the difference."

In her own soft, quiet way, Brooke seems to have caught up with herself and to know exactly where she is going, including the four years at college for which she is saving the money she earns.

It's true that none of her peers have told her that she's beautiful, "but I've sometimes felt that some of the boys would like to if they knew what to say."

Brooke and her mother, Teri, live in an East Side apartment with two cats and Teri has a black jeep in which she drives her daughter to her jobs and picks her up.

They leave today for a ranch in Arizona, where they will visit for a few weeks. Brooke won a medal for best all-around athlete at a summer day camp a few years ago, but riding a bucking bronco was not included.

from the NEW YORK POST, July 15, 1977

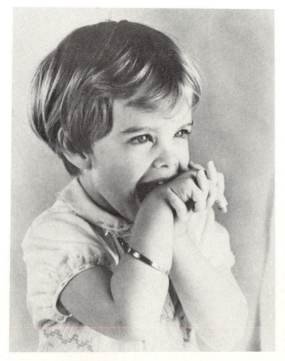
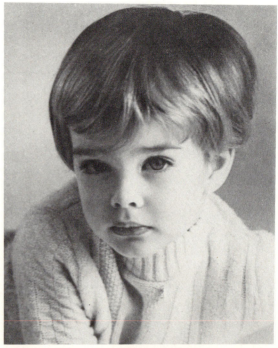
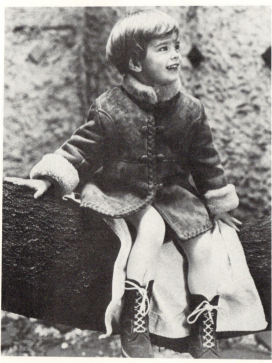
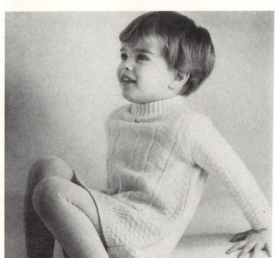

BROOKE SHIELDS

Birthday 5-31-65
Age Range 2 - 4
Eyes   - Blue
Hair   - Blonde

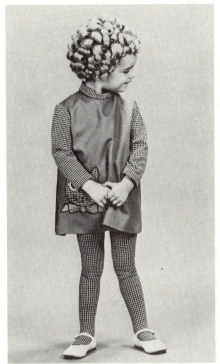
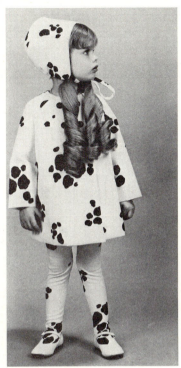

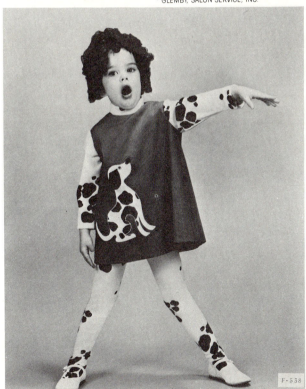

F-538   Dalmatians never had it so good.

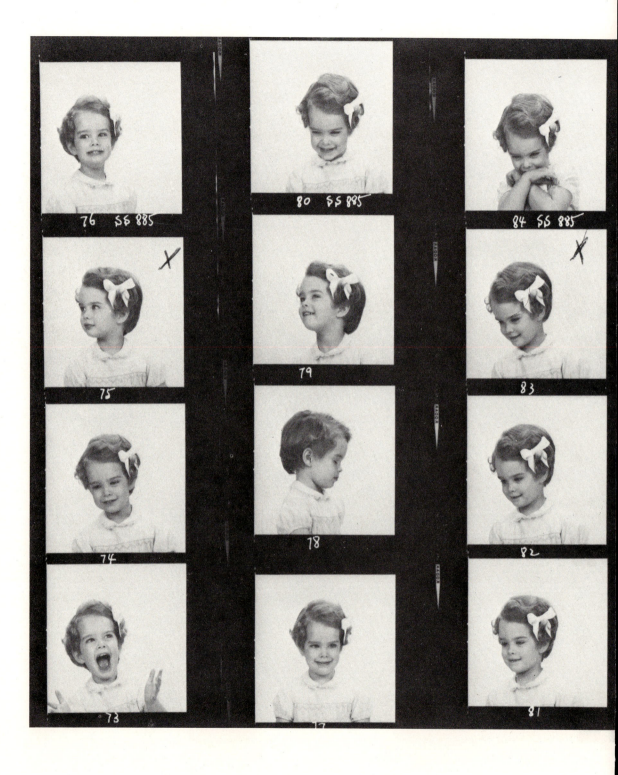

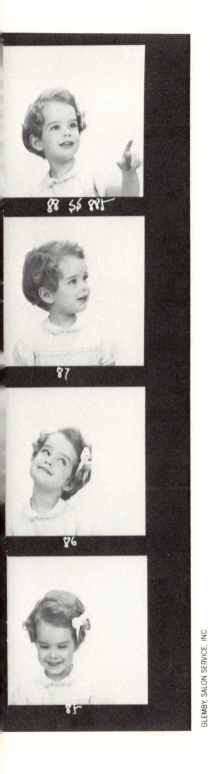

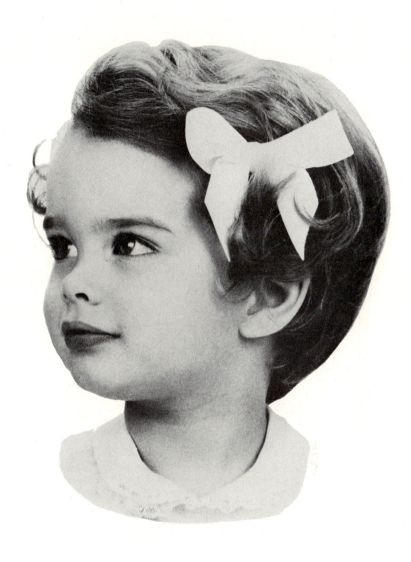

THE GEM & I
Oh thinker of fidelity,
Pretty baby, you're a child;
Who conquers with maturity,
All adventures, however wild.
Liño Ruiz, 1977

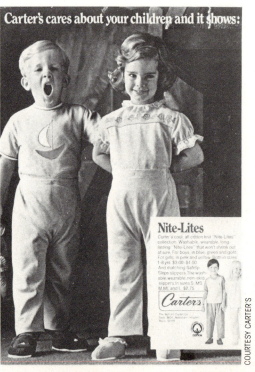

Carter's cares about your children and it shows:

Nite-Lites

Carter's cool, all cotton knit "Nite-Lites" collection. Washable, wearable, long-lasting "Nite-Lites" that won't shrink out of size. For boys, in blue, green and gold. For girls, in pink and yellow. Both in sizes 1-6 yrs. $3.00-$4.00. And matching Safety-Steps slippers. The washable, wearable, non-skid slippers, in sizes S, M5, M, M6, and L. $2.75.

Carter's

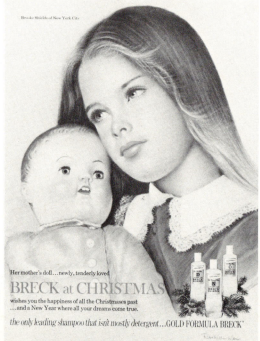
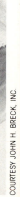

Brooke Shields of New York City

Her mother's doll...newly, tenderly loved

BRECK at CHRISTMAS

wishes you the happiness of all the Christmases past ...and a New Year where all your dreams come true.

the only leading shampoo that isn't mostly detergent...GOLD FORMULA BRECK

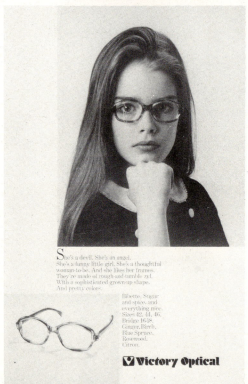

She's a devil. She's an angel.
She's a funny little girl. She's a thoughtful woman-to-be. And she likes her frames. They're made of rough-and-tumble zyl. With a sophisticated grown-up shape. And pretty colors.

Bibette. Sugar and spice. and everything nice. Sizes 42, 44, 46. Bridge 16-18. Ginger, Birch, Blue Spruce, Rosewood, Citron.

Victory Optical

VICTORY-OPTICAL

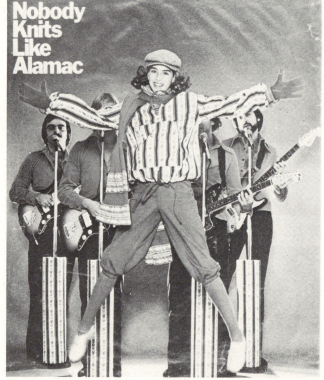

Nobody Knits Like Alamac

WEST POINT PEPPERELL

What's the right way to take a bandage off?

A cut heals better when it's kept covered.

But most kids don't know how to change a bandage when it's time to put a fresh one on.

When they take an old bandage off the wrong way, they can pull the cut open.

Here's the right way.

Gently peel back both sides at the same time so there isn't any pressure on the cut.

Now go ahead and put a fresh one on. And keep it on until the scab is gone.

If you don't keep it on, the scab can get knocked off.

And then you have to start healing all over again.

Getting hurt once is bad enough.

It heals better when it's covered.

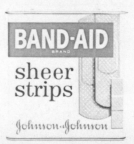

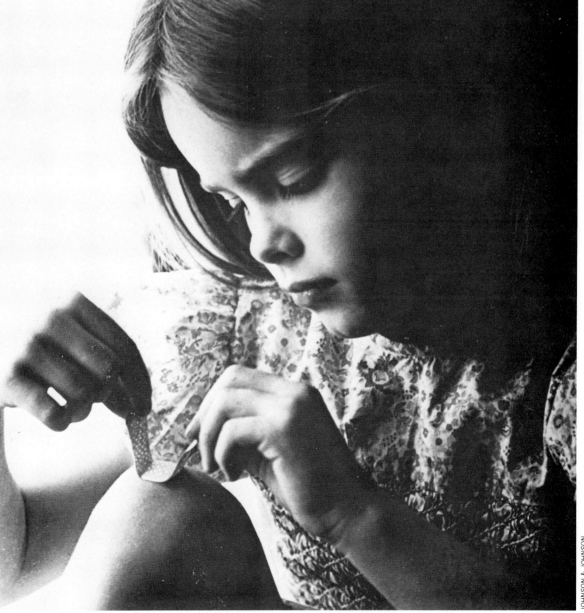

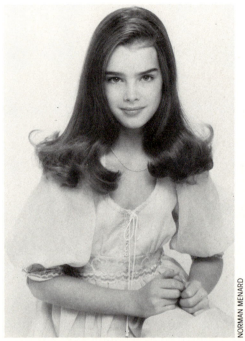

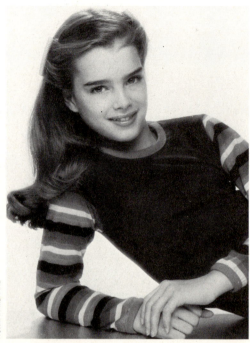

Test shots for the Breck Ad

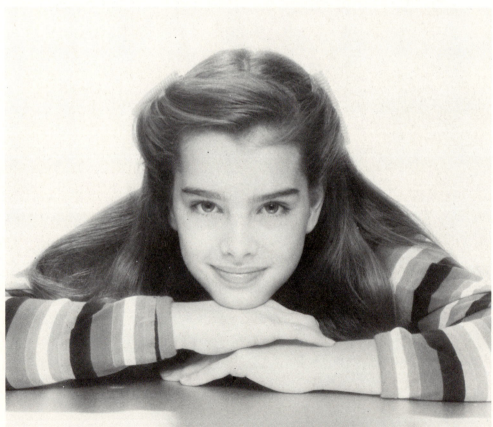

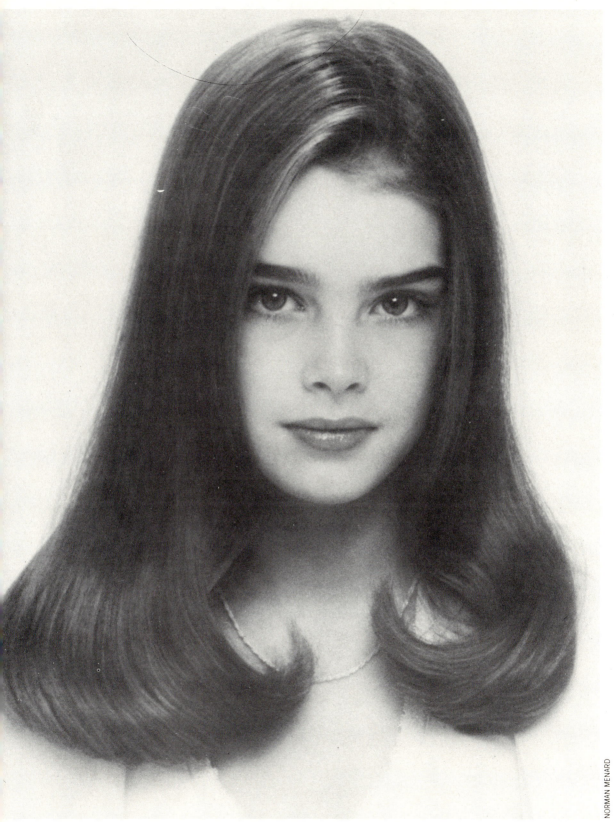

I worked
from 7:30
in the morning
to 9:15
in the night.
The photographer
said curses
and all ways
pointed me
out and
said things
like we
don't need
your two sense,
that took care
of her and
I will throw
you off the set
if you don't
stop pulling
on your dress.
But the only good thing
about the job was that
I got to collect

shells and dip my feet
in the bay.
On the way home I played.
When we arrived in N.Y.C.
and were
getting off
the van
I found
a dollar.
The driver
of the van
said it
was probably
his
because
I asked him.
The job
was
in someplace
called
Gay Hampton
or something
like that.

June 11, 1975

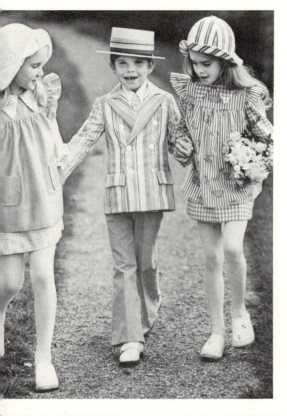

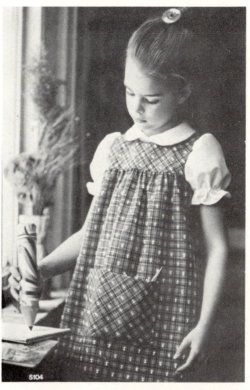

5104

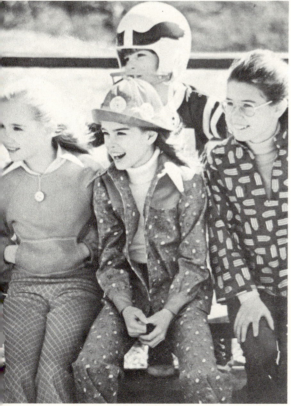

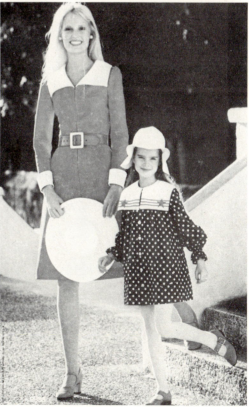

SIMPLICITY PATTERNS CO., INC. GEORGE BARKENTIN, PHOTOGRAPHER

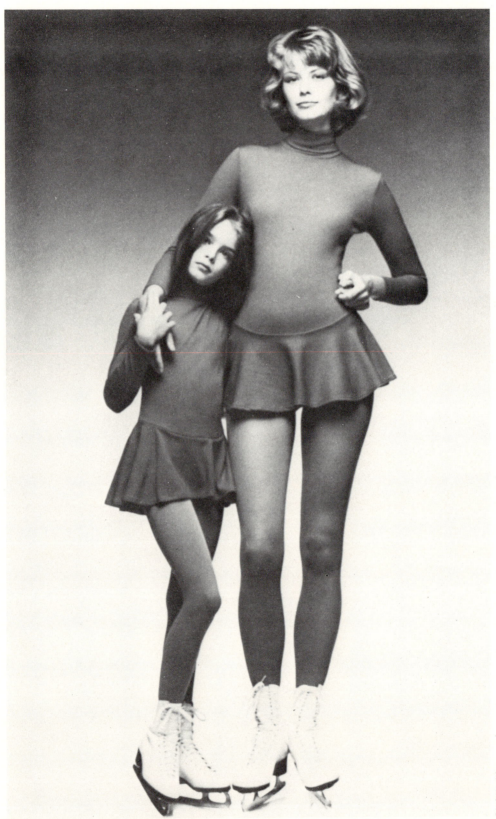

Her name is Charlie. It's hard to iceskate on plastic.

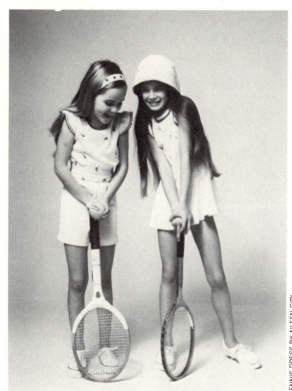

TENNIS DRESS BY AILEEN GIRL

Kelly Ridge with me.

DANCING

When I dance upon the floor
my mind goes whirling like a silver ball
rolling down a hill,

My feelings come out and I'm in a dream
world floating up and up on a cloud,

But when the music stops
I slowly come down as my
cloud fades away.

I am in the middle of my good morning world.

November, 1976

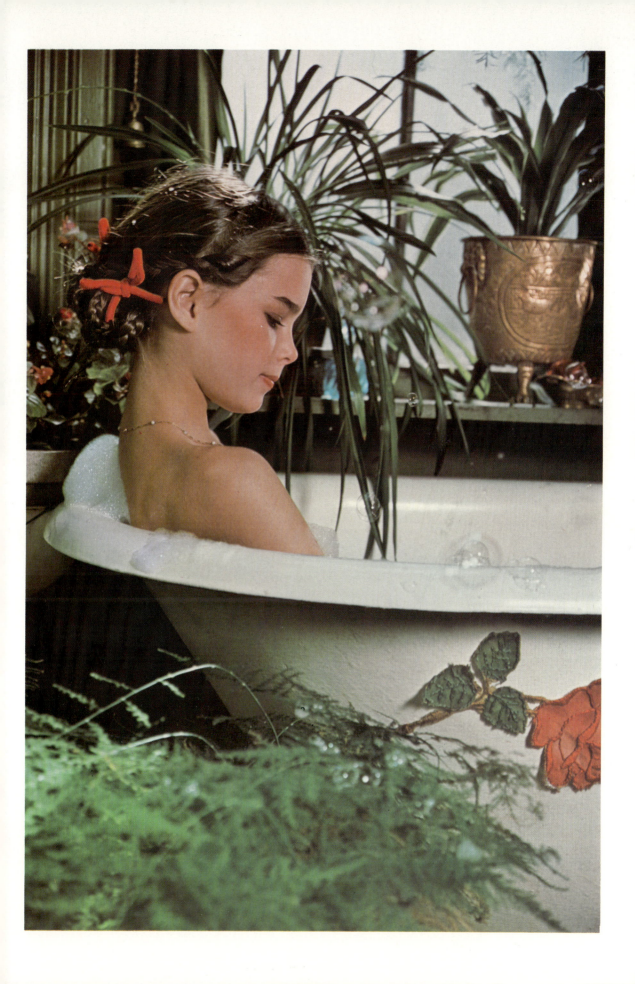

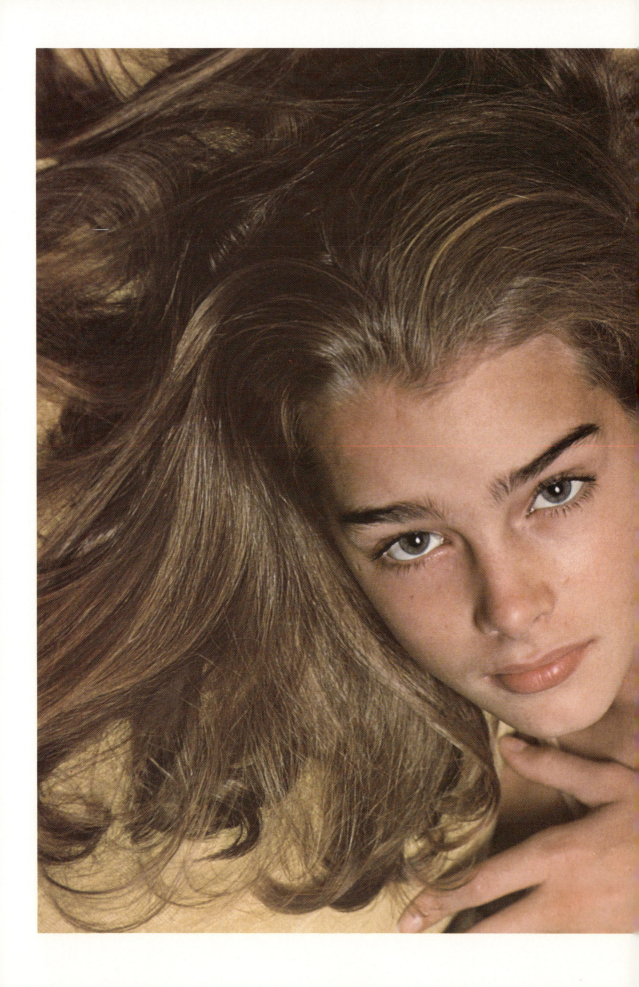

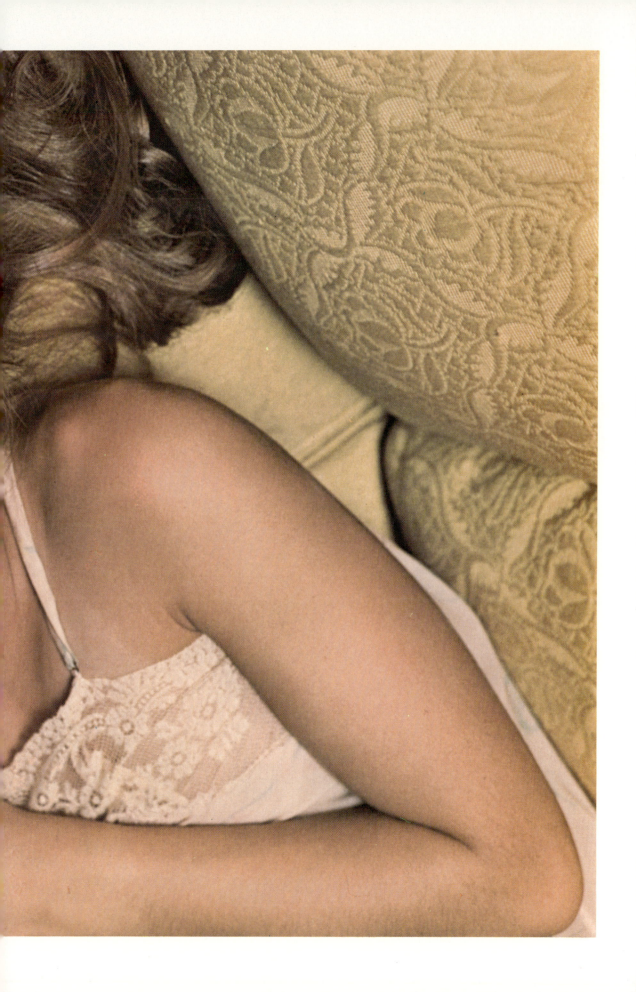

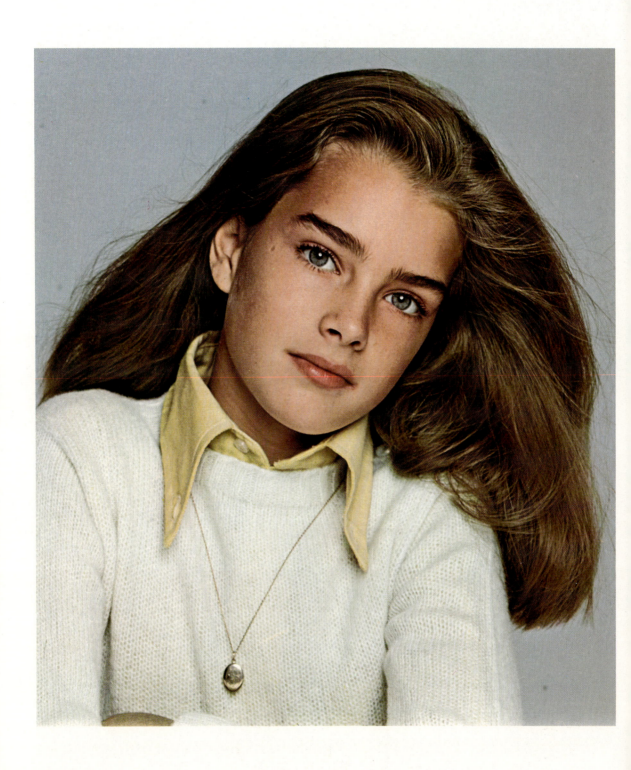

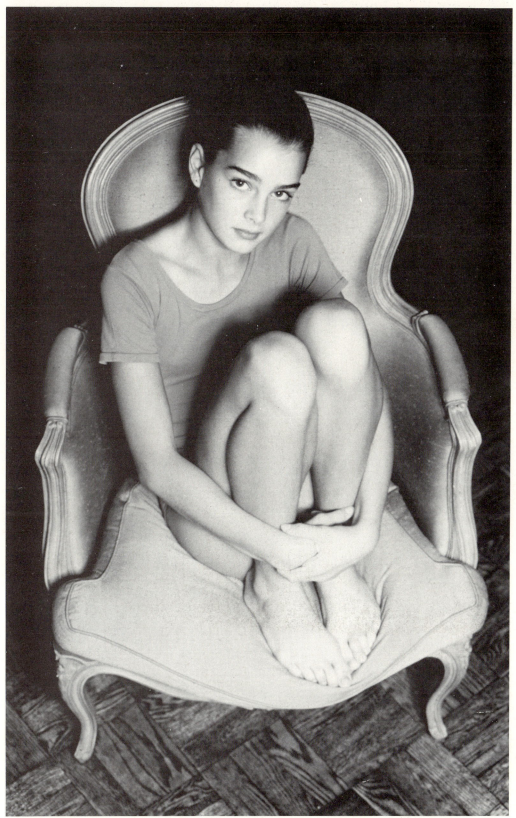

APACHE MAGAZINE. TADASHI ENDO, PHOTOGRAPHER.

Here I am in Molly Lee's blue chair.

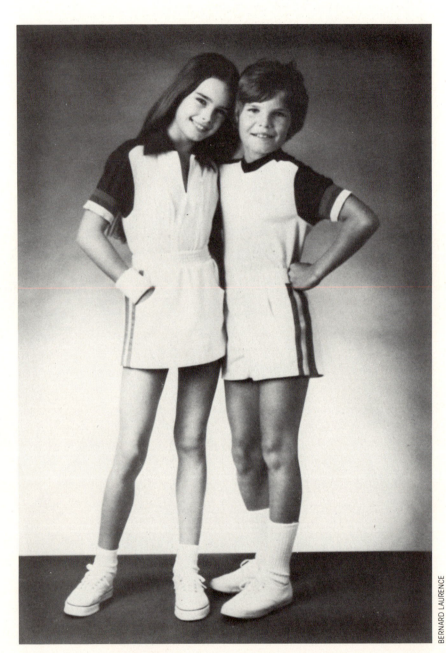

Neal Bodack and I, for Head Sportswear.

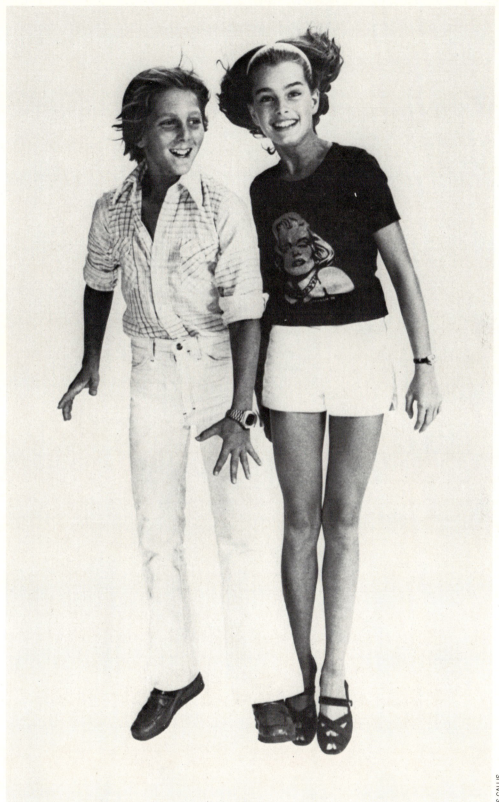

Whee! We just landed parts in MORNING, WINTER AND NIGHT.

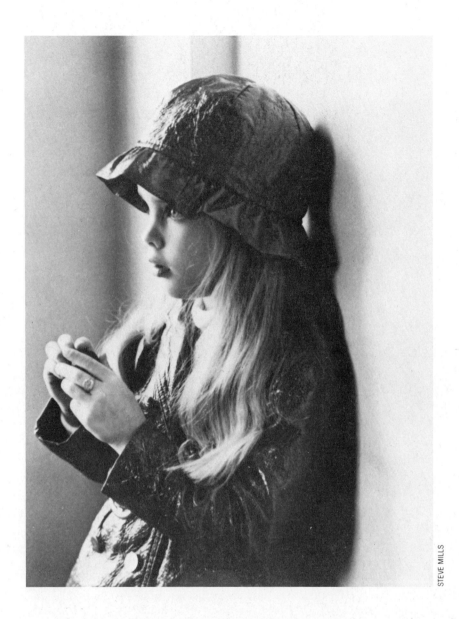

STEVE MILLS

This bird lives in a bird's nest in California
    and eats bread and bird seeds and worms.

Once upon a time there was a little frog
and his name was Sam
and the little frog had a friend
and his friend was named Sam, too
and they loved each other very much.

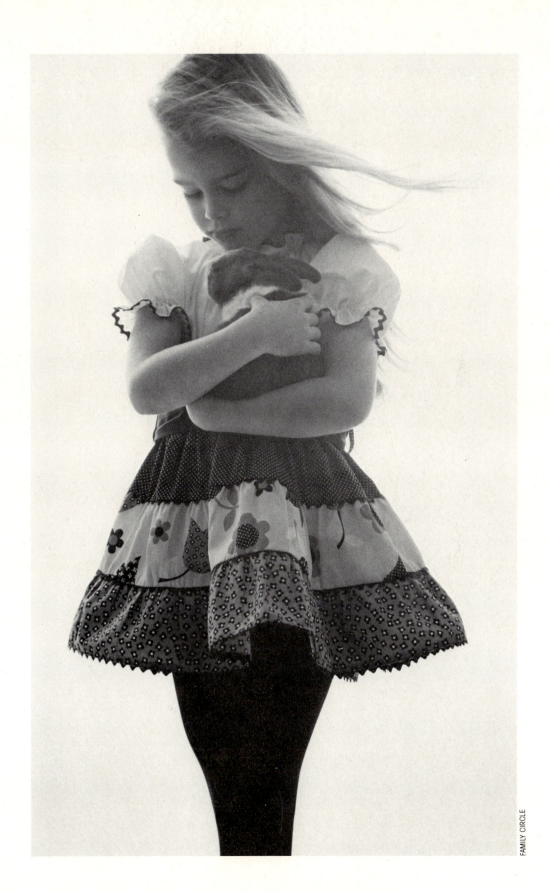

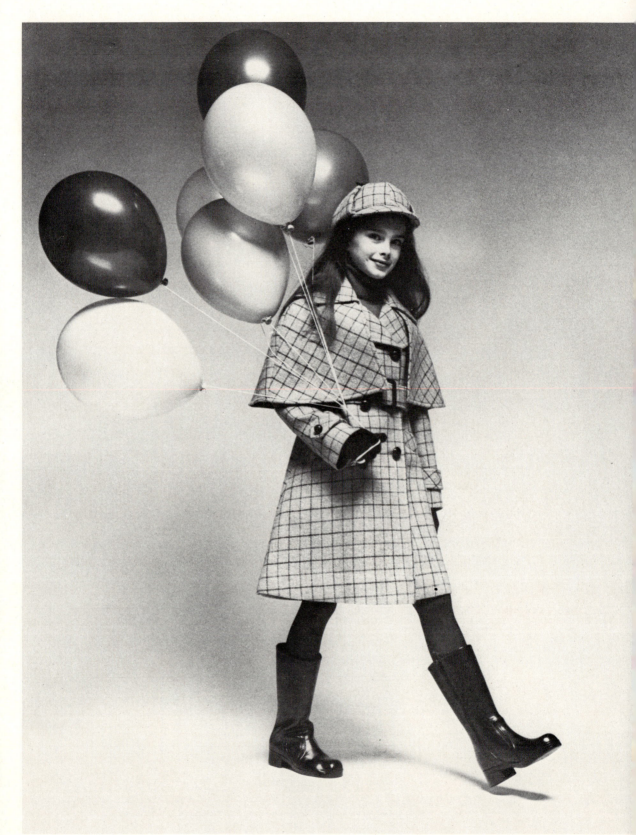

GIMBELS. BARBARA KAPLAN, ART DIRECTOR; CLAYTON ADAMS, PHOTOGRAPHER.

BALLOONS

Balloons can make someone
                          Happy
Especially when given to a
                          Child
But when blown away
                    sadness enters.
                    November, 1976

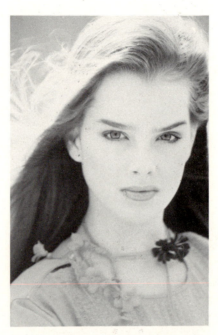

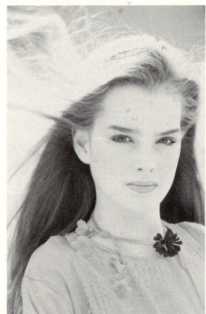

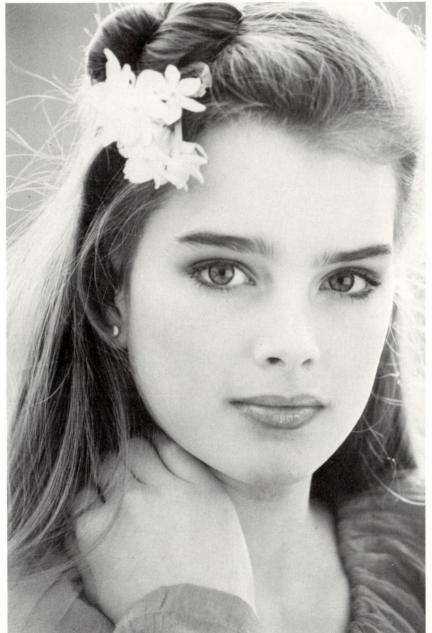

GEORGE BARKENTIN, PHOTOGRAPHER, FOR SEVENTEEN MAGAZINE AND USED BY PERMISSION

Thank you, George Barkentin.

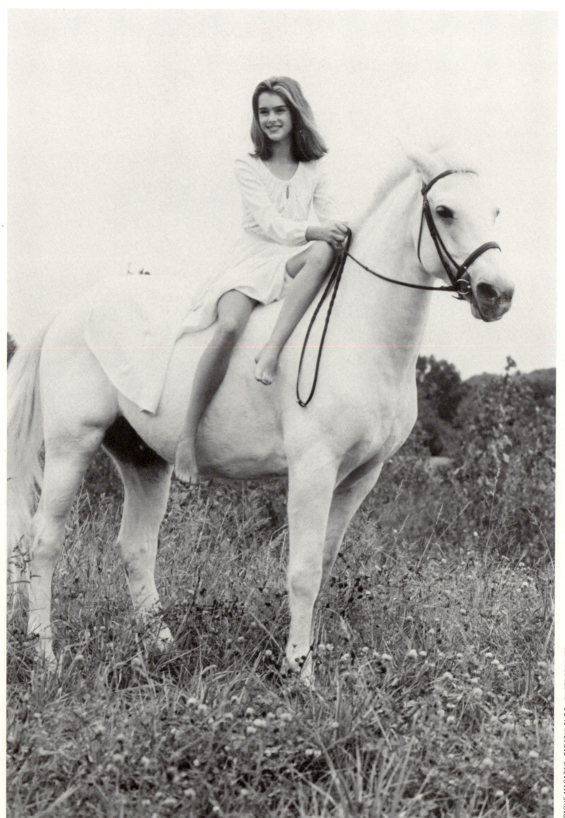

In the country . . .

APACHE MAGAZINE. TADASHI ENDO, PHOTOGRAPHER

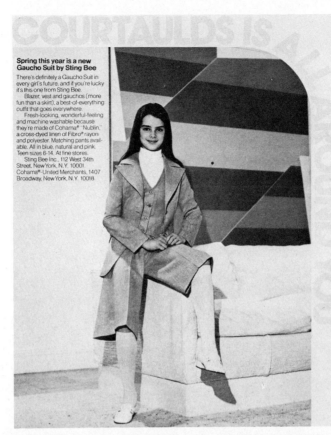

**Spring this year is a new
Gaucho Suit by Sting Bee**

There's definitely a Gaucho Suit in
every girl's future, and if you're lucky
it's this one from Sting Bee.

Blazer, vest and gauchos (more
fun than a skirt), a best-of-everything
outfit that goes everywhere.

Fresh-looking, wonderful-feeling
and machine washable because
they're made of Cohama® "Nublin,"
a cross-dyed linen of Fibro® rayon
and polyester. Matching pants avail-
able. All in blue, natural and pink.
Teen sizes 6-14. At fine stores.

Sting Bee Inc., 112 West 34th
Street, New York, N.Y. 10001.
Cohama®-United Merchants, 1407
Broadway, New York, N.Y. 10018.

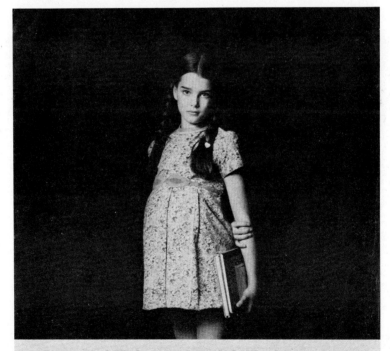

First period, Math. Second, English. Third, Parenthood.

*"Keeping Up With Youth" by Pamela Swift
February 1, 1976 issue*

She's 12. She's evidently pregnant.
And thanks to Philadelphia's humane
approach to girls between the ages of
12 and 17 who are infanticipating,
she still goes to school.

A special school. With regular scho-
lastic courses, plus family management,
menu planning, etc. Parade readers

already know the news, even though it
won't make headlines in their local
papers. That's the appeal of Parade.

*Incisive reporting about world-shat-
tering news, little people with big
problems (like that poor kid), even
Hollywood chatter.*

As an advertiser, you should take

more than a scholarly interest in
Parade.

Learn why it's on the honor roll of
111 leading newspapers with something
like 41 million readers. All it takes
is a collect call to (212) 953-7650.

Parade. It isn't very heavy, but it
carries a lot of weight.

parade

It wouldn't be Sunday without a Parade.

AUTOGRAPHS

Hi, my name is Maryann Gilligan. I am known on my block for the girl with the most autographs. Everybody thinks I show off about them but I know I don't.

My parents Mr. and Mrs. Sam Gilligan are famous skaters. They are constantly in competition, so we travel alot.

Once we drove to the state of Washington for one of my dad's competitions. It took several hours to get there but I didn't mind. When we arrived I heard Dorothy Hamill was going to be in competition, so I asked my mom if I could go to see her and she said, "Yes."

We were at the rinks about an hour and a half before the competition began. I saw the rink and it had a straight red line in the middle dividing the rink in two parts. One side was for speed skating and the other was for the competition of that day. Then I caught sight of Dorothy Hamill fastening her skates, I was so excited that I started running toward her. My mom stopped me and said, "Don't bother her now, she is busy." As she stood up I saw she had a nice figure and she wasn't too broad.

Finally the competition started. All the girls went before Dorothy. Then it was her turn. When she started skating so beautifully and so steady that she didn't make one mistake. I was sure she was going to win the gold medal.

When the last measure of music was over Dorothy came off the ice and sat down. Then I walked over to her and shaked, I mean shook her hand and asked if I could have her autograph. She said, "All right."

At home I told everybody what had happened and they thought I was showing off again. I know deep inside, I wasn't.

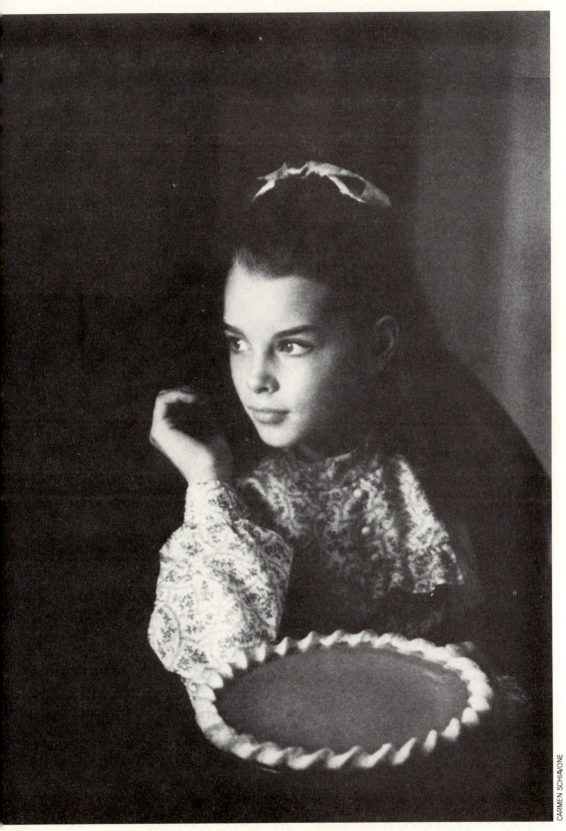

I don't even like pumpkin pie!!!

If I were a pair of shoes I'd try not to lose my heels.

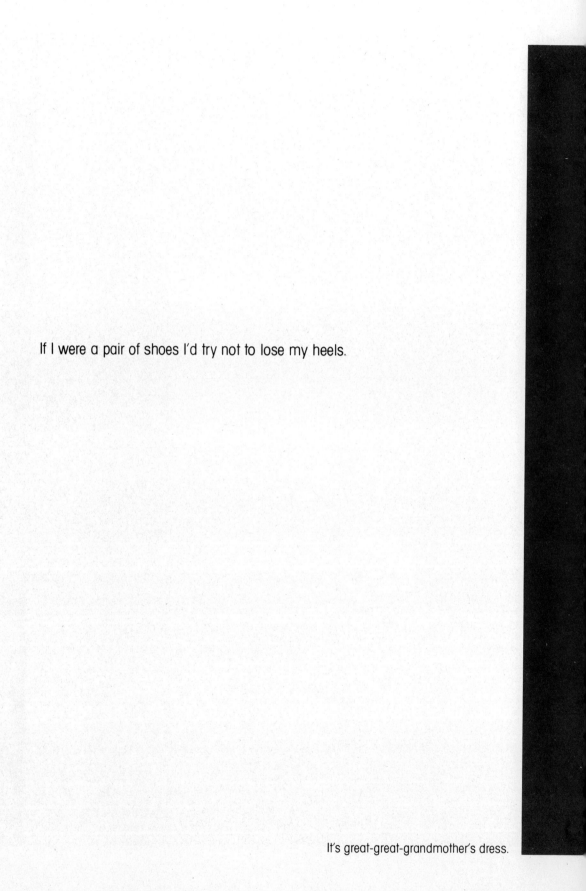

It's great-great-grandmother's dress.

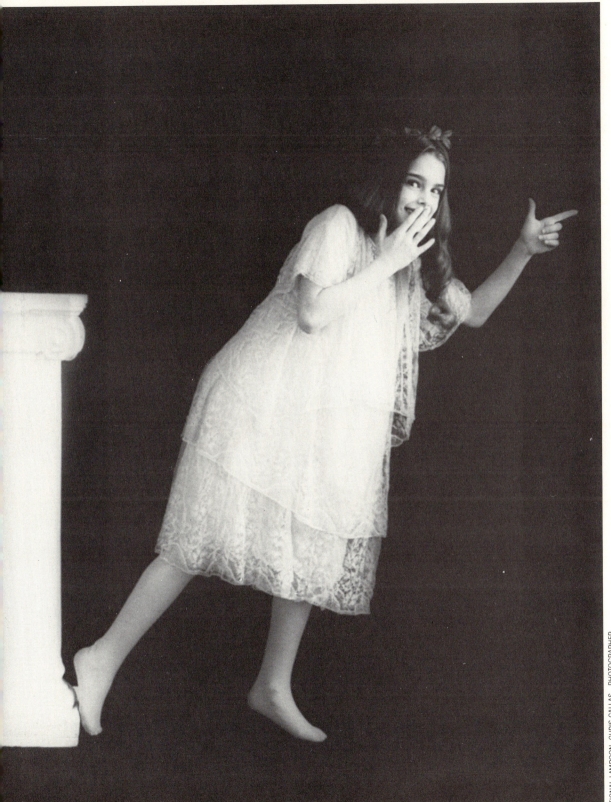

NATIONAL LAMPOON CHRIS CALLAS. PHOTOGRAPHER

When I was sixteen and dropped out of school I needed a job. I wasn't sure if I wanted to be a guard at a <u>building</u>, or a <u>buyer</u> in a <u>guitar</u> store.

I have a <u>guinea pig</u> who had babies. I felt <u>guilty</u> because I couldn't keep them. I had many buyers for them. Two were <u>guests</u> of a party I had gone to some weeks ago. I had sold two to two of my friends that said that they would take good care of them because they had a <u>guide</u> book on animals.

The guinea pigs gave me a good idea because Halloween was coming soon so I decided to <u>disguise</u> myself to look like them. I <u>guess</u> I will be the biggest guinea pig in town.

Last night I had a dream that my <u>guardian</u> angel said that she was a good <u>builder</u> and built me a building with my name on it and then <u>guided</u> me into it and said that I could call her any time I needed <u>guidance</u>.

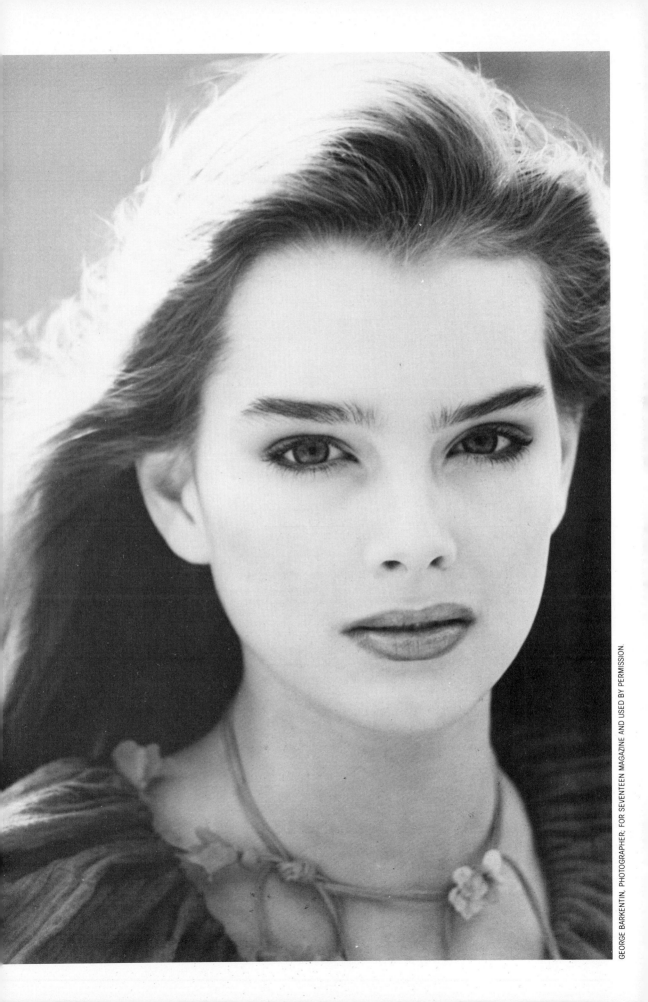

Do you believe that I have my own dressing room that has my name on it. Isn't that fun?

I'm having my hair curled and yesterday the lady who is curling my hair now, took a handful, made it damp, took a razor blade and ran it down my head from about ½ way in the middle of my head . . . to make my hair thin . . . so it will hold a curl. YUK!

Paramount wanted to pluck my eyebrows but neither my mother or I would let them do it. NO WAY!

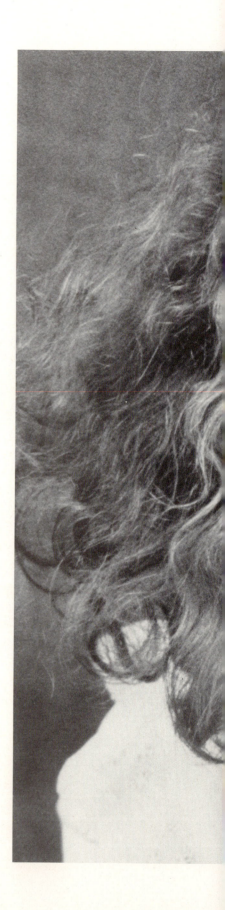

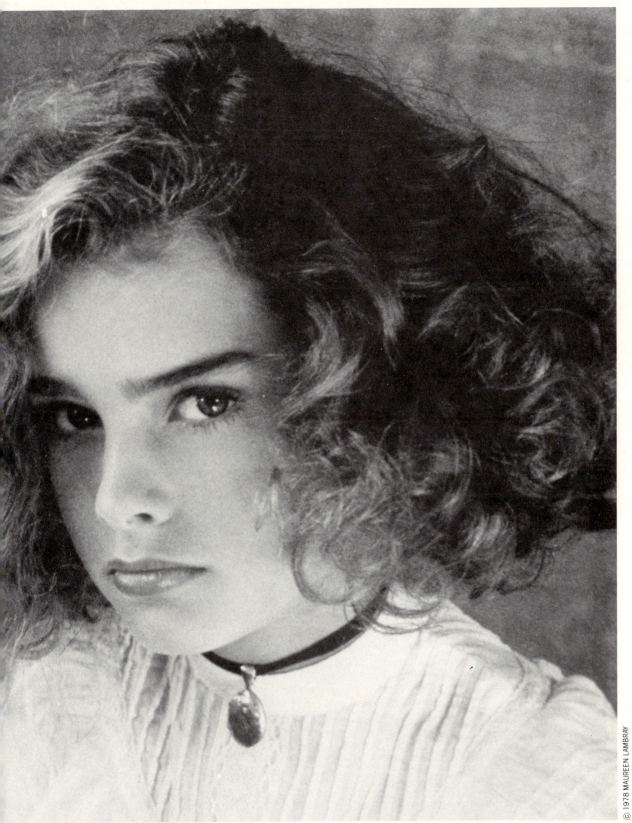

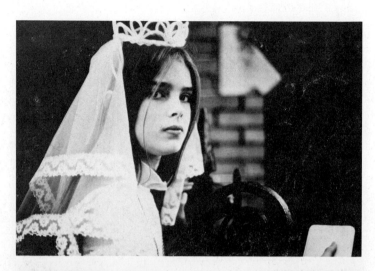

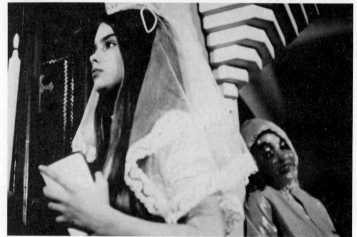

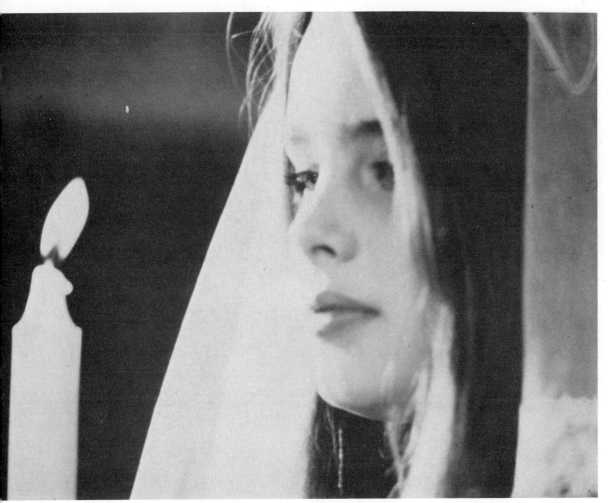

FROM ALICE SWEET ALICE, A FILM PRODUCED BY RICHARD K. ROSENBERG AND DIRECTED BY ALFRED SOLE. AN ALLIED ARTIST RELEASE.

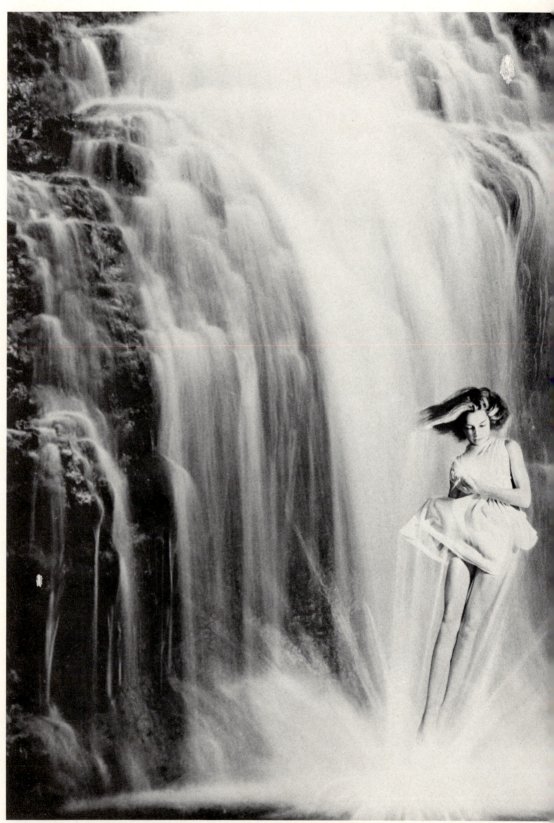

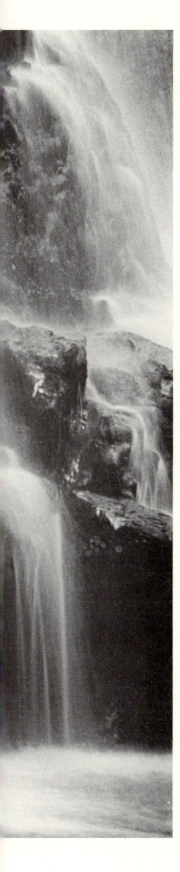

Happiness is a swimming pool
    a pretty flower
    pretty grass
    ice cream
    a new drive-in movie
    getting up early in the morning
    a smile
    silly people

We shot the album cover the day of the black-out in NYC.

World's youngest sex symbol?

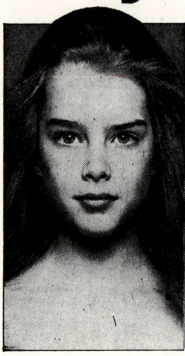

**11:45 PM
"WEEKEND"**
She has the body of a child and the face of a gorgeous woman. She's 12-year-old Brooke Shields, soon to be seen as a prostitute's daughter in a major motion picture.

This and other features tonight on "Weekend." Lloyd Dobyns reports.

4 **N** NBC News

PETER POOR, WEEKEND

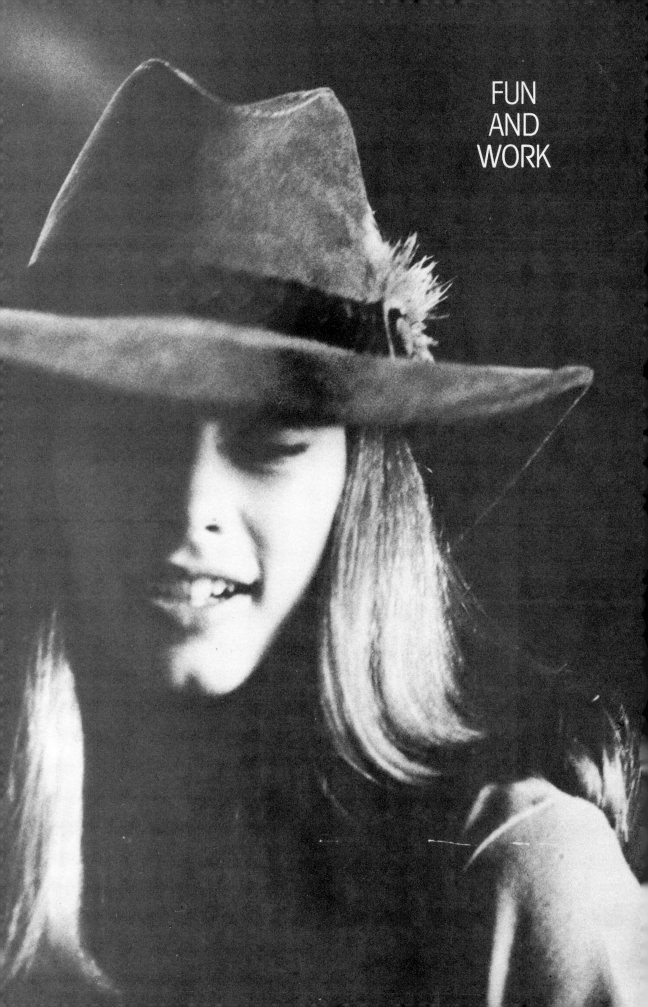

FUN
AND
WORK

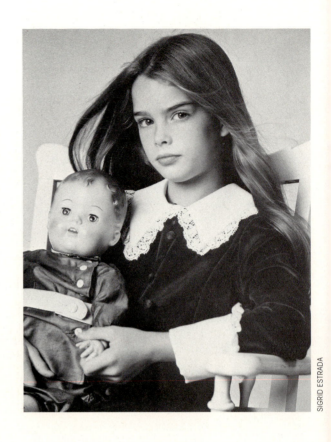

THE DOLL

My name is Brooke. One day I went to a store looking for a birthday present for my niece. On one of the shelves there was a doll like a musician and the <u>expression</u> on the doll's face was <u>precious</u>. There was a little tag that said <u>caution</u>, breakable but I knew that my niece would take good care of it.

The man at the store had a French <u>accent</u> that I liked very much.

Then I bought my niece a box of <u>delicious</u> candy. On the box there was an <u>artificial</u> flower.

I remembered that my niece liked to go ice skating so I took her to the rink. In the middle of the rink there was a big <u>glacier</u>.

You had to have <u>patience</u> to skate with my niece because she is not a very good skater and always falls down.

For dinner we went to a restaurant called National Autocar. It was called that because there was a big ancient car in the middle of the restaurant.

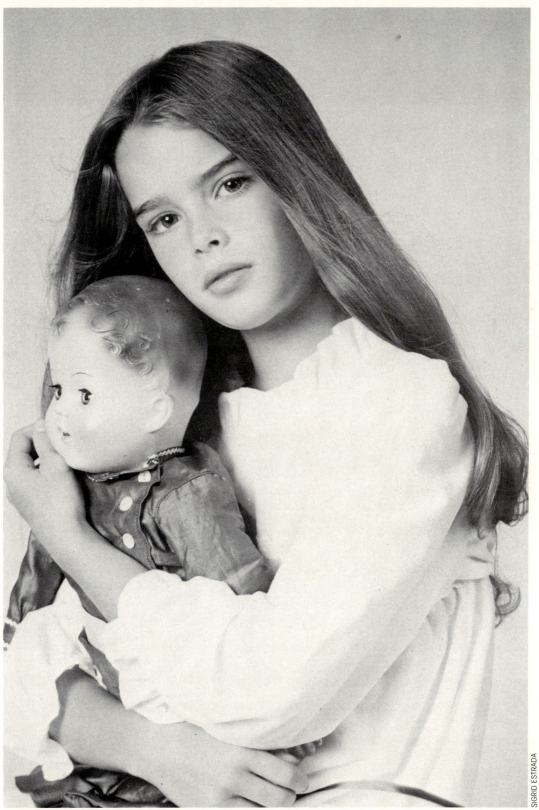

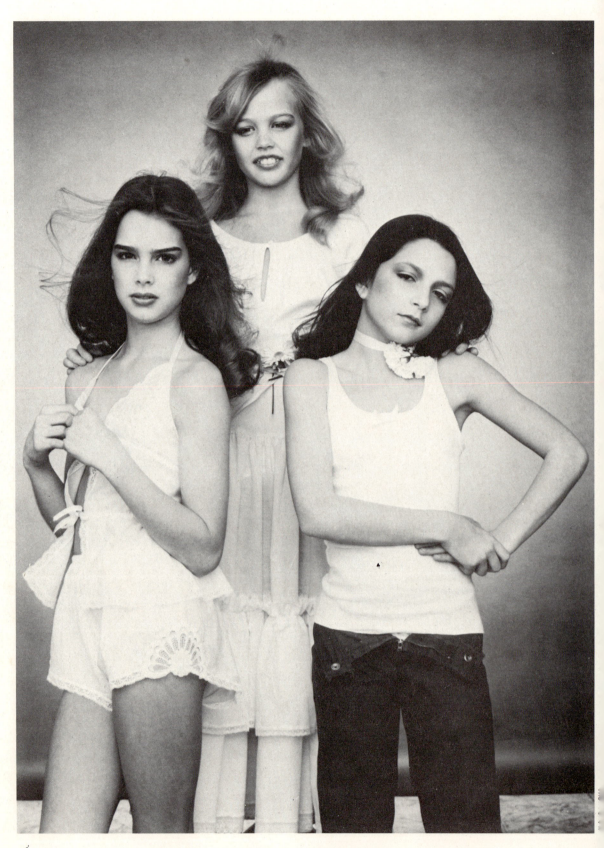

Janet Rooney and Alicia Dale and I playing "Charlie's Angels."

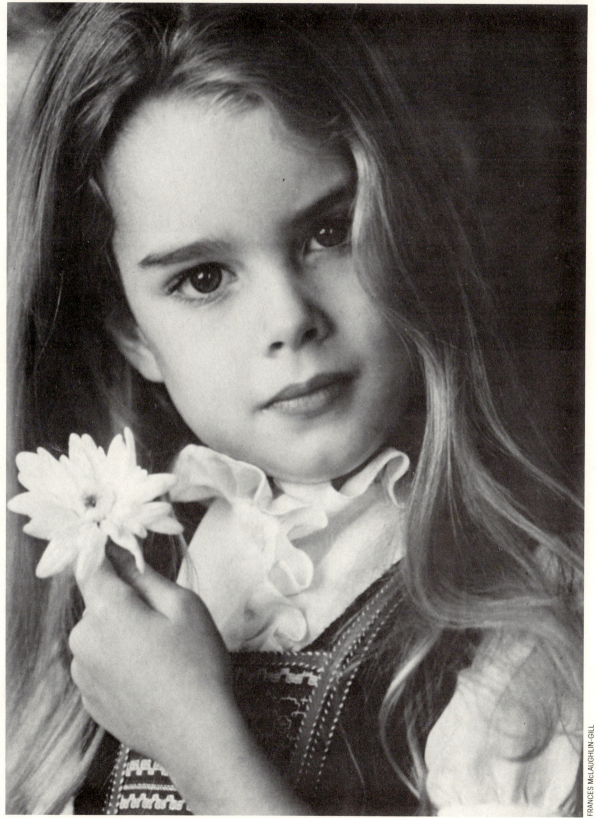

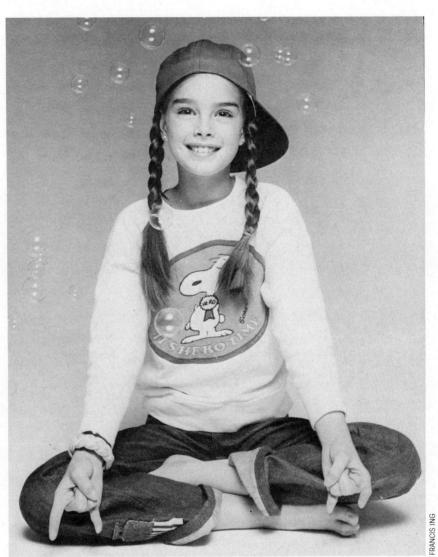

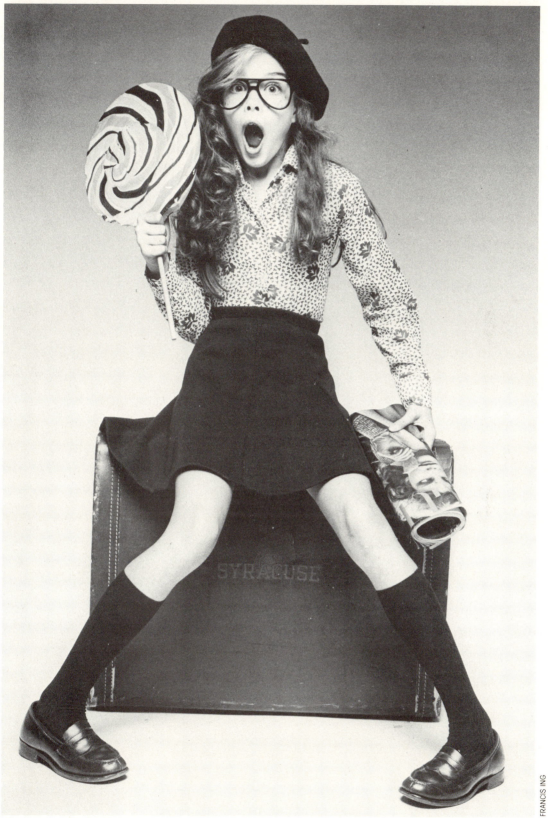

THE WICKED WAR

When I went to war I traveled six thousand miles in a boat. I practically starved because there was little food. When we disembarked the captain walked up to me and said, "You are now at war!"

I was selected to go to tent B. On the way I was surprised how many wounded soldiers there were. In my tent I arranged my gear and then stretched out on my cot. The tent was not crowded but it was a little stuffy.

In my spare time I took two pieces of paper and traced a picture of a rifle and sent it to my wife.

After the first six months I wanted to go home.

When I got home I bought the kids a little something. They squeaked with joy and paraded around the room.

My wife said that I shouldn't have bought them something but I winked at her and said it was alright. The kids also tracked around the room.

I was ashamed I neglected to bring my wife something but she was so happy to see me it didn't matter. I admired the way she took it.

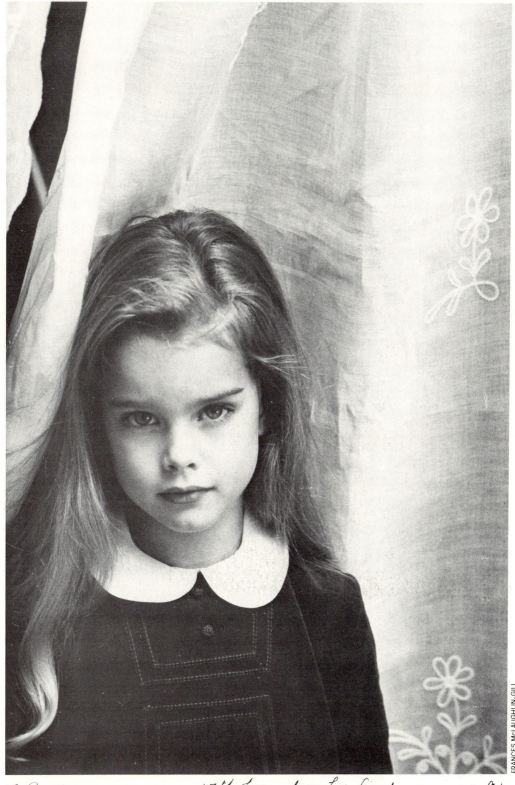

To Brooke,

with love from her friend —
Frances McLaughlin-Gill

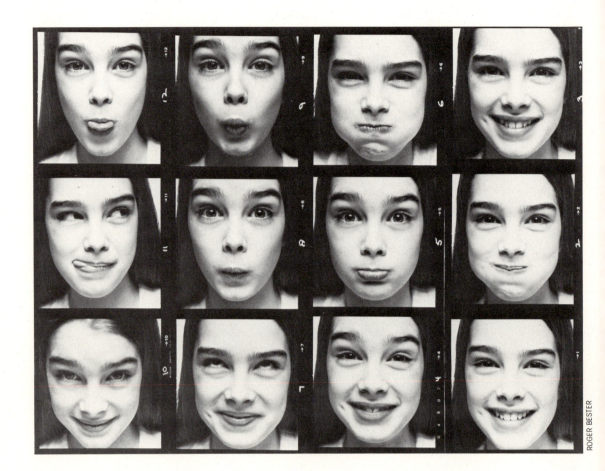

ROGER BESTER

GREED

Many years ago the Gods sent an oracle that said, ANYONE THAT SHOWS THEIR GREED WILL BE PUNISHED IN SOME WAY. Among the people who heard the oracle was a little boy named Dimi. Dimi had a little dog he loved very much. He couldn't do enough for his dog. The dog never appreciated anything and always wanted more. Dimi came from a poor family, so there wasn't much food. Dimi would always share what he had with his pet.

Once a year all the town people would gather to have a big feast. Each family would contribute something to eat or drink. They would contribute something that they worked hard for all year. Dimi's family offering was a huge piece of meat.

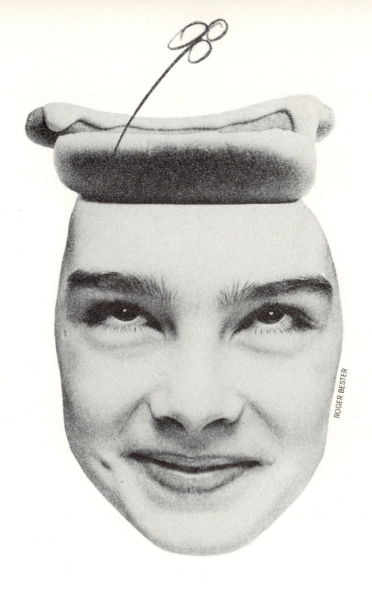

ROGER BESTER

The day of the feast was here. All the tables were set with all kinds of goodies. While Dimi was playing with his friends, his bad dog stole the beautiful piece of meat. The dog took the meat to a nearby pond and rested for a while. Much to the dog's surprise he saw another dog in the pond looking up at him with even a larger piece of meat in his mouth. Not realizing that it was his own reflection, the greedy dog lunged at the other dog to steal his meat, and lost his own piece.

Just as the oracle had predicted, it doesn't pay to be greedy.

February, 1975

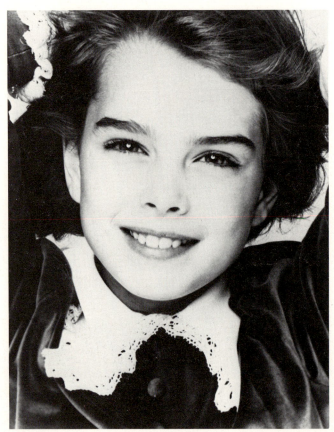

DAVID STEINBERG

Say:
OOCSHALA SHANGWALA LA LA LA
LA LA LA LA HELAMANY CHELAMANY
CELA BELA DELAMANY
while saying these words
turn around 3 times
then look in the mirror
and make a wish.

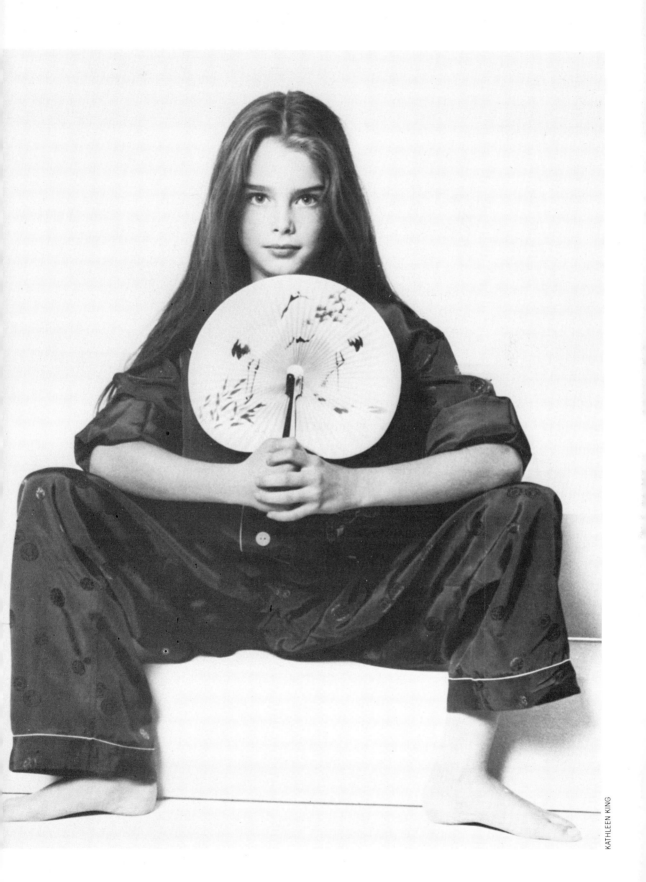

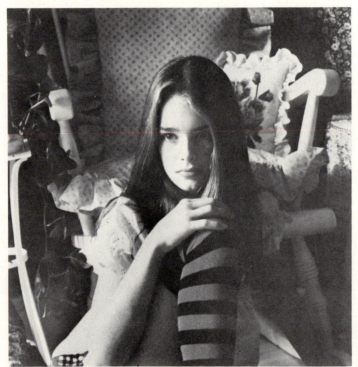

STEVE MILLS

It was the Merry Bicentennial Xmas.

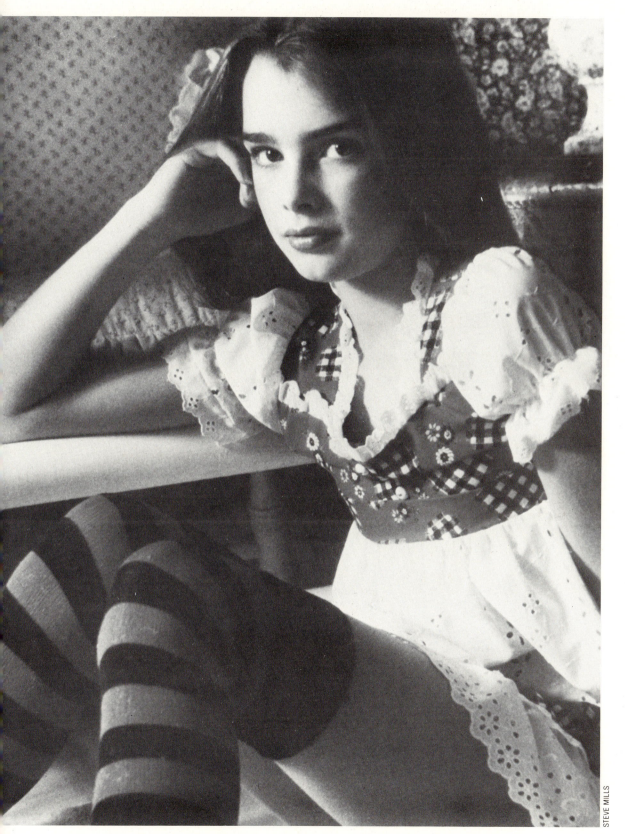

My friend Poppy was the stylist.

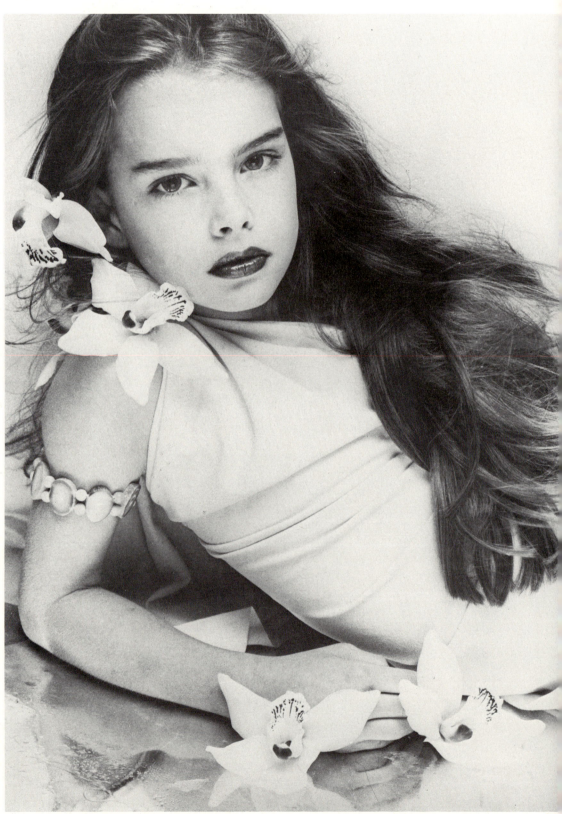

FRANCIS ING

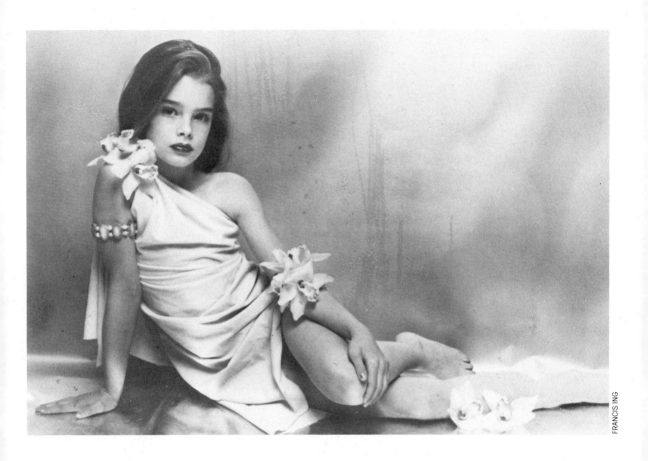

FRANCIS ING

SIN

Sin it may be,
To think such thoughts
That come from within.
Hell's heart (if there be one)!
But I know that God
Our Father will forgive us
From his heart,
which definitely exists.

November, 1976

I love my cat
I love my bunny
I love my cat
     for she's my
     honey.

1973

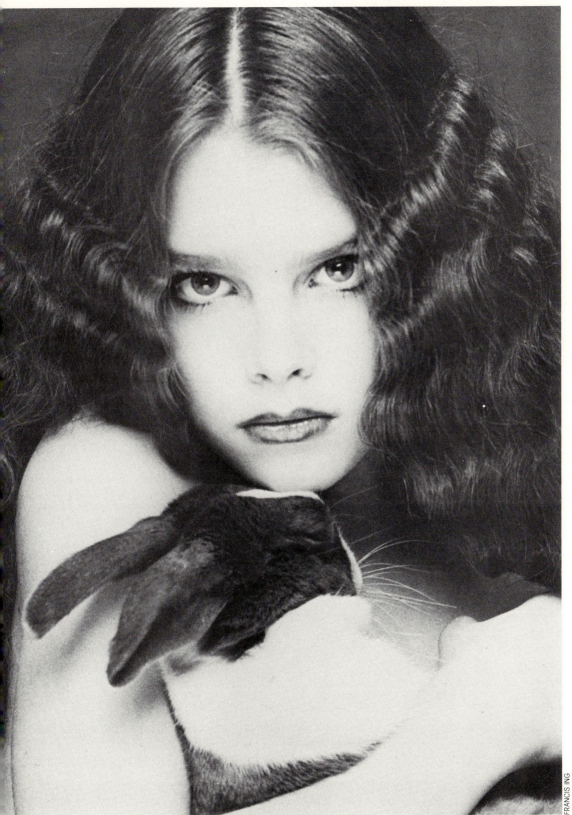

THE STORY OF
MADAME LASLOW AND ISABEL

The story starts with a lady named Madame Laslow who thinks she is very smart. Although she wasn't, she still thought that she was.

One bright morning in the middle of the night Madame Laslow got up to fight with the lady next door. The lady's name was Isabel. The two of them had grumbled about something the other day. The two were the ugliest people on the block. Whenever Madame Laslow or Isabel would look in a mirror, the mirror would break. And when they would sing a high note the building would shake.

Well, getting back to the fight. Madame Laslow put on her boxing gloves and suit and met Isabel at the corner. When the fight began the score was first one to one, then one to two, then two to three. Isabel won. She had three.

Madame Laslow got mad that when she arrived home she was thinking of a trick to pull on Isabel. She thought for an hour, finally she had an idea. Halloween was coming so she decided to dress up as Isabel and rob the biggest bank in town.

Halloween morning finally came. She put her duds together. She looked exactly like Isabel from head to toe. Last but not least she put in her green false teeth, that looked exactly like Isabel's.

Off she went to the First National Bank where she held them up and stole all the money she could get her hands on. When she arrived home she quickly undressed and waited for the kids to come trick or treating. Needless to say ugly Miss Laslow went to bed smiling.

The next day the newspaper headlines read UGLY ISABEL ROBS FIRST NATIONAL BANK, and is captured and put in jail for 20 years.

That is the story of Madame Laslow and Isabel.

THE END
1974

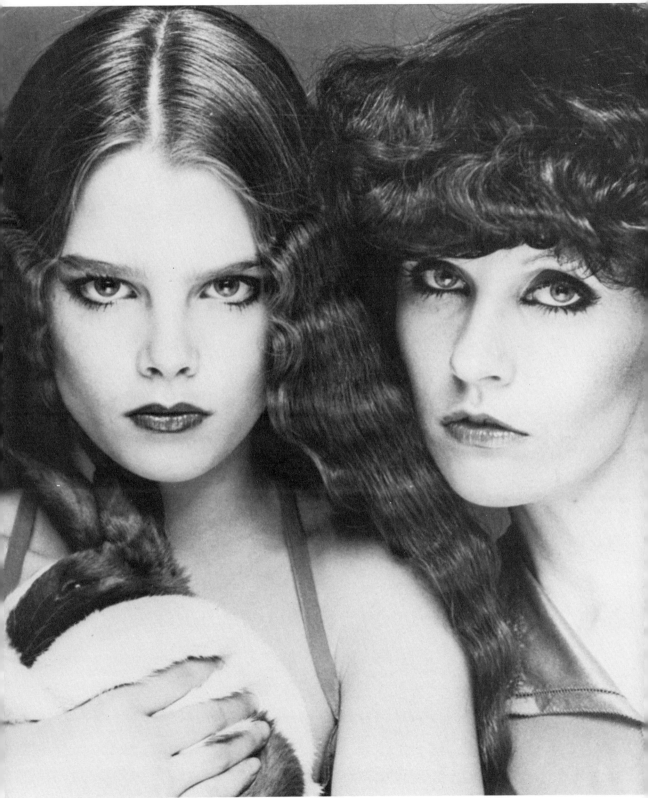

FRANCIS ING

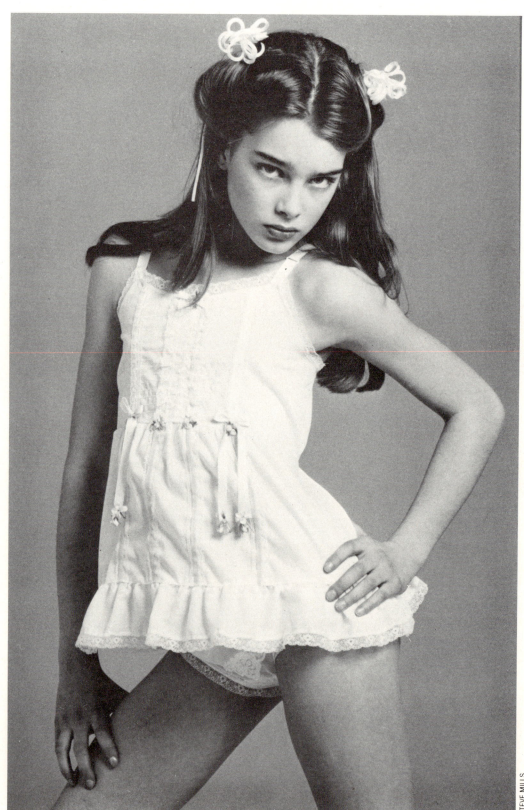

"She posesses a quantity
of that undefinable whatever,
perhaps detached awareness."
            — Steve Mills

FIRE

Quick,
        as the blazes of
fire go climbing into the
deep blue of the sky,
        as the eyes of the
people are fixed on the
blaze,
        then the last sound
of the crackling fire is
the beginning of silence.

November, 1976

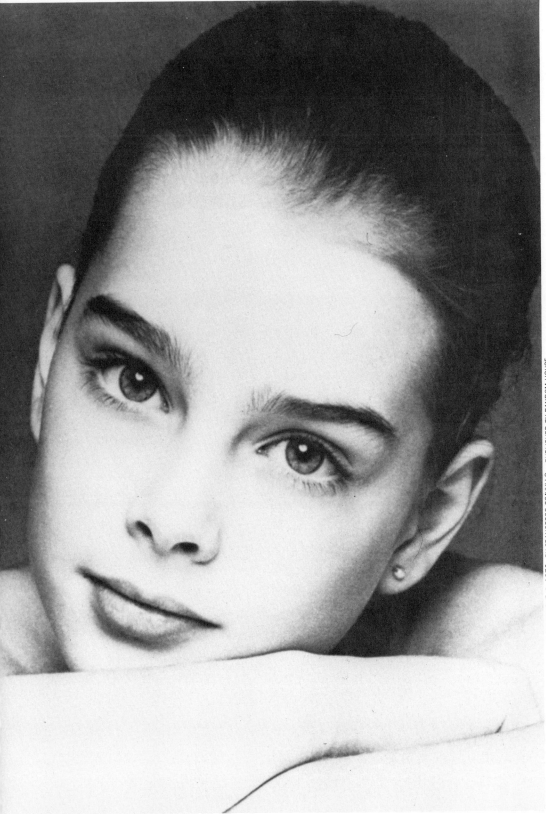

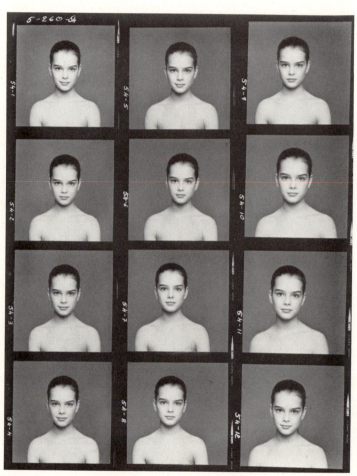

NOT AN ORDINARY ANGEL

Hi, my name is Samantha Loving, otherwise known as Sam or Sammy Loving. I am going to tell you about an angel or my angel also named Samantha Loving or otherwise known as well you know. Anyway it all started one Saturday morning while watching T.V. By the way, I was watching Happy Days and all of a sudden my room became very very bright and a small figure appeared right in front of me. I can't explain what she (I believe she was a she, I mean, you know what I mean) looked like but she was kind of short, her hair was a rusty brown and she was wearing jeans and a tee-shirt that said, IT'S COOL UP THERE. She was the first to speak. "Gimme some skin," she said. And, of course I did what any ordinary person would do. I gave it to her.

"Nice pad you have here," she exclaimed.

"Who are you, how did you get here and what do you want," I questioned.

"Oh, how could I forget, I am your private, secret, nice, beautiful, thoughtful and sweet . . ."

"Get on with it," I interrupted.

"Well," she said. "I am your angel and I am to stay with you until you reach the age of fourteen, when you will be old enough to take care of yourself properly."

"I'm old enough now," I insisted.

"Trust me, the dude up there sent me and he knows his business," she said pointing her finger up to my ceiling. I agreed.

"You're no ordinary angel," I said not being able to help myself.

She apparently liked that because she said, "Thank you." Then she said, "Let's have some chow and then I will tell you what I am to do with you." While munching on an English muffin she said, "Oh, I almost forgot, down here on earth I am visible only to you, because I am only your angel."

After chow as she called it we went to my room and she explained that she was here to help me grow more capable of myself.

Well, because I am eleven, the first year was alright but if I went to parties she would always be there. Other than that she was really fun. We would play games and people would stare at us (really me) because they could not see her and it looked funny because all of a sudden the ball would stop in mid-air because she would catch it. I thought to myself, she would make a great magician's assistant. She could make things rise up in the air. We really became good friends, as a matter of fact she said I was her best earth friend.

The last year was great. We had so much fun because by that time it was summer. It soon ended, the last year was over and I really felt mature. It was a sad sad good-bye. It was quick and she gave me a medal that I earned from growing up.

I'll always miss her and I'll think of her often. I still have the medal though it also, is invisible, which makes it more secret.

Early 1976

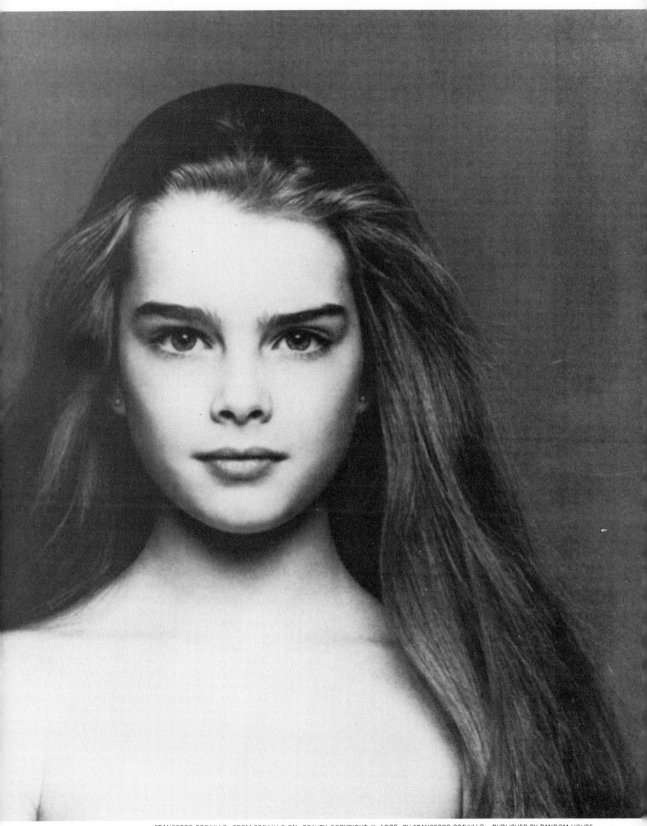

I guess it's because I look twenty-one in my first warm coat.
Fur just makes me feel so fantastically sexy.
You know what I mean.

MANHATTAN

Manhattan is a place with
        lights that never quit
Dresses that cost alot and
        Some that only cost a bit
Swarming with restaurants and
        Stores down the block
As people stare at Times Square's
        big clock.
                        October, 1975

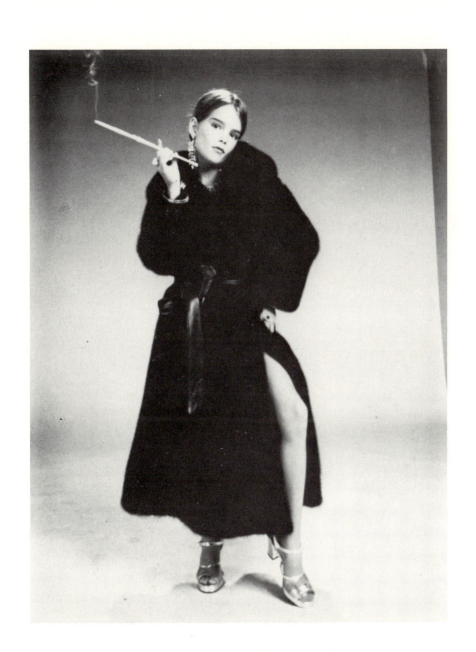

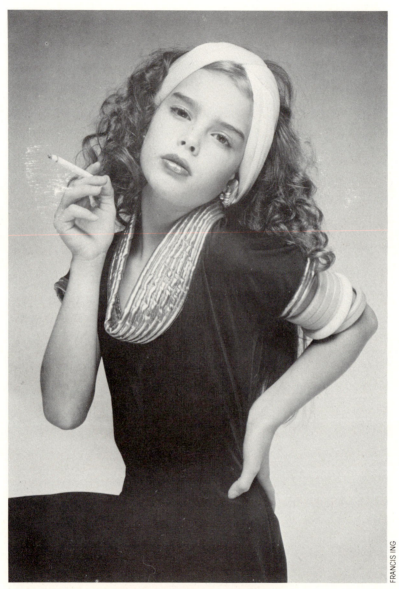

FRANCIS ING

"It's only a role. I am an actress."

CALIFORNIA

A different world
    as it will be
    is all so strange
    to you and me.

The hills go up
    and the hills go down
    the sun so bright
    it makes you frown.

The roads are long
    the sky is blue
    it is full of excitement
    just
       for
          you.

          California
          Summer 1977

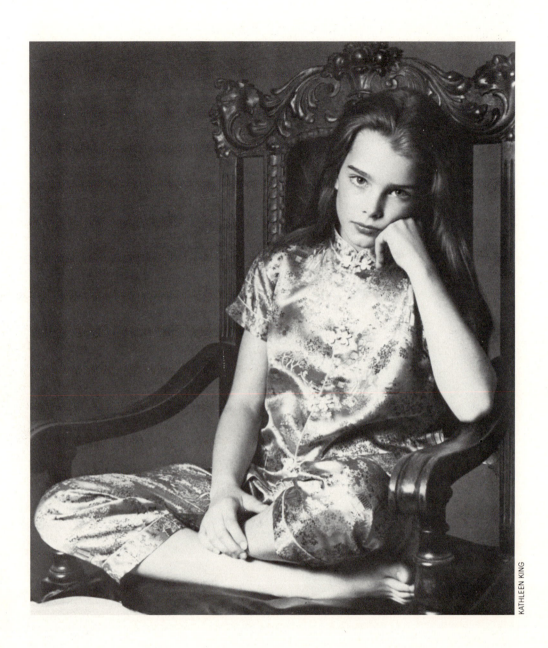

KATHLEEN KING

MUSIC

Music is a kind of thing
    that makes you really want
To sing and when you sing
    you sing out loud
Then when you're finished
    you feel proud.

1975

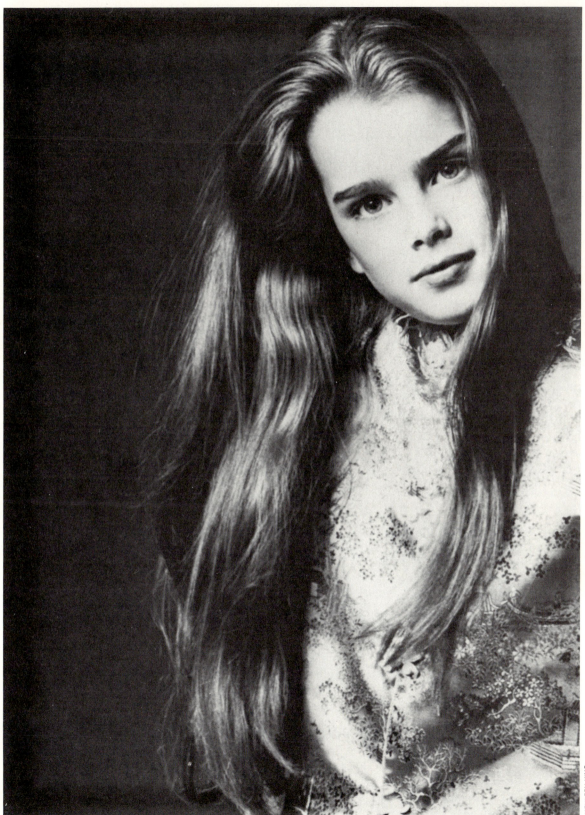

KATHLEEN KING

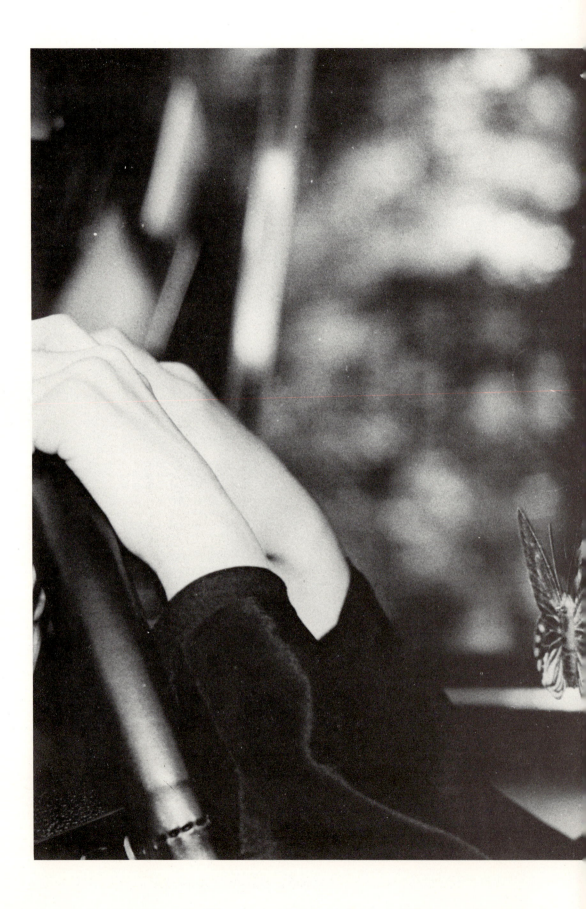

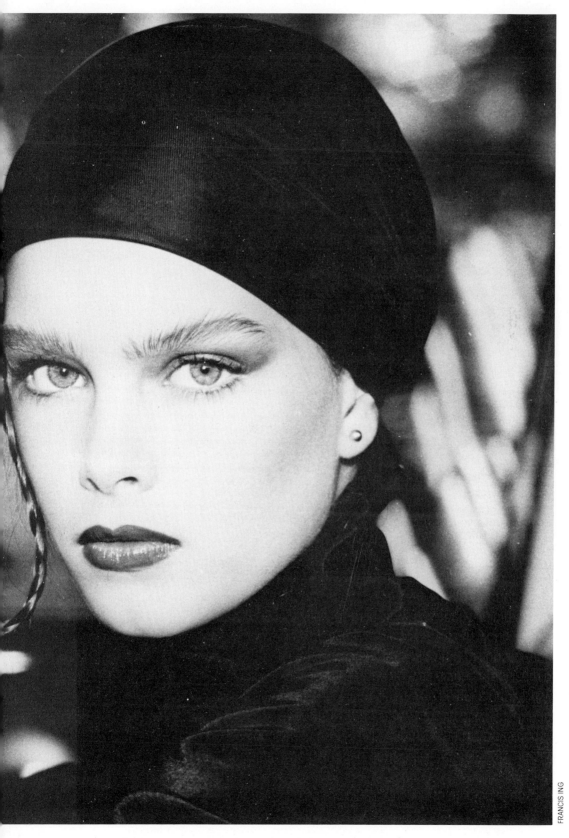

FRANCIS ING

Sometimes I feel like a million bucks because I look like, a million bucks.

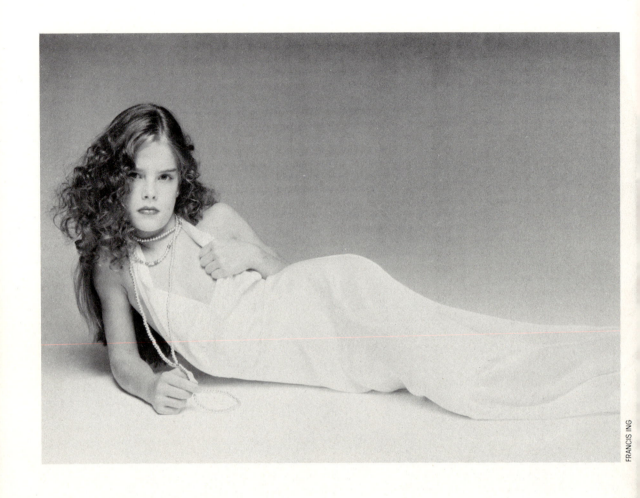

FRANCIS ING

STAINED GLASS WINDOWS

Stained glass windows are
a beautiful sight because
When the sun shines in they
look so pretty and bright
People look at them in delight
when they find out a
Beautiful sight is seen.
1975

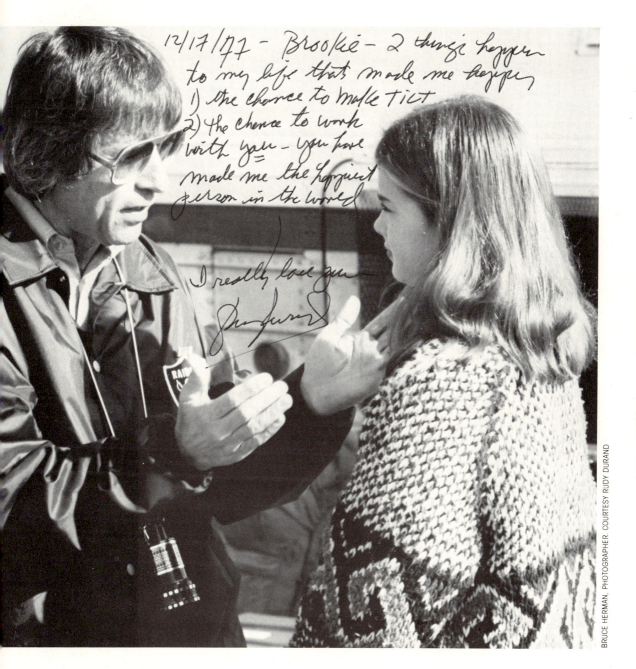

12/17/77 - Brookie - 2 things happen
to my life that made me happier
1) the chance to make TILT
2) the chance to work
with you - you have
made me the happiest
person in the world

I really love you -

[signature]

With Rudy Durand, director, writer and producer of my new movie, TILT.

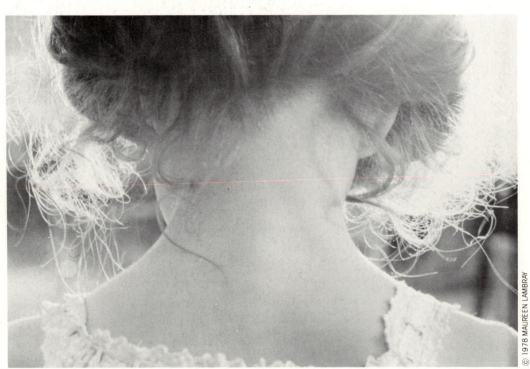